UNSEEN

UNSEEN

HOW I LOST MY VISION BUT FOUND MY VOICE

A MEMOIR

MOLLY BURKE

ABRAMS PRESS, NEW YORK

Copyright © 2025 Molly Burke

Jacket © 2025 Abrams

Published in 2025 by Abrams Press, an imprint of ABRAMS. All rights reserved. No portion of this book may be reproduced, stored in a retrieval system, or transmitted in any form or by any means, mechanical, electronic, photocopying, recording, or otherwise, without written permission from the publisher.

Library of Congress Control Number: 2025934749

ISBN: 978-1-4197-7788-2
eISBN: 979-8-88707-457-3

Printed and bound in the United States
10 9 8 7 6 5 4 3 2 1

Some names and identifying characteristics have been changed. Some dialogue has been re-created.

Abrams books are available at special discounts when purchased in quantity for premiums and promotions as well as fundraising or educational use. Special editions can also be created to specification. For details, contact specialsales@abramsbooks.com or the address below.

Abrams Press® is a registered trademark of Harry N. Abrams, Inc.

ABRAMS The Art of Books
195 Broadway, New York, NY 10007
abramsbooks.com

ABRAMS is represented in the UK and Europe by
Abrams & Chronicle Books, 1 West Smithfield, London EC1A 9JU
and Média-Participations, 57 rue Gaston Tessier, 75166 Paris, France.
abramsandchronicle.co.uk | media-participations.com
info@abramsandchronicle.co.uk

I dedicate this book to the followers who have stood by me through it all—thank you for always giving me the grace to change, learn, and grow. It's been an honor to share my twenties with you, no matter how messy at times.

And to every disabled advocate and activist who has come before me, thank you for paving the path I now have the privilege of walking. Your efforts have not gone unnoticed and have made an immense difference to people like me. I vow to continue to put in the work to fight for the rights we all deserve. The biggest gift I could receive is knowing I've impacted the lives of future generations the way you have impacted mine.

One way in which I'm trying to do this is with this very book. I'm choosing to center the disability community with every choice I've made, from the cover design to the font selection. While most books use a serif font, which is deemed easier to read for the average person, I have chosen Atkinson Hyperlegible, a sans-serif font that is more legible for those who are low-vision or have print-reading disabilities, like Dyslexia. For the same reason, I've chosen to use **boldface** text instead of using *italics*, which also helps. The font size and spacing, along with the color of the paper used, were all taken into consideration to make this a comfortable reading experience for my community.

CONTENTS

AUTHOR'S NOTE	v
PROLOGUE	1
INTRODUCTION	5
TIME TO GET TO WORK	14
BUT DAD, I DON'T WANNA GO TO COLLEGE	27
THIS IS WHAT DREAMS ARE MADE OF	37
A MOMENT OF SILENCE	48
I'LL DO ANYTHING	58
THE MOUSE THAT BROKE THE CAMEL'S BACK	63
LOVE BOMBING, GASLIGHTING, AND NEGGING, OH MY!	70
FALL FROM GRACE	81
RED FLAGS WAVING	89
FADE TO BLACK	99
A FOUR-LEGGED FRIEND	106
FAKING IT	116
SEEING THE FUTURE	120
SHE'S GOING TO BE A STAR!	126
I STILL WON	131

CONTENTS

BLINDBEAUTY07	141
SUBSCRIBE	149
A SQUEAKY-CLEAN CALL	155
NO ROOM FOR A GIRL LIKE ME, HUH?	161
THE GUY WITH THE GLASSES	167
IF THE SHOE DOESN'T FIT	174
AMERICA'S NEXT TOP ROLE MODEL	180
DUMBO	184
"SHORTY" GIRL PROBLEMS	194
PRETTY GIRLS WALK LIKE THIS	198
HATERS GONNA HATE	204
YOU CAN'T BUY EQUALITY	208
LAST NAME BURKE	214
THE FACE OF BLINDNESS	225
ALL FOR ONE AND ONE FOR ALL	229
LOUDMOUTH	236
EPILOGUE	247
GLOSSARY	251
ACKNOWLEDGMENTS	257

PROLOGUE

I was anxiously standing backstage on the set of **The Daily Show**, eagerly anticipating hearing Trevor Noah announce my name. White cane in hand, I was beginning to regret my choice in footwear. 6.1-inch bubble-gum-pink Versace heels weren't exactly practical, but I've always been a girl to put fashion before function, and either way, it was too late now.

The day before, I had sat in my New York City hotel room discussing my options on the phone with producers. I could either begin my live-to-tape interview onstage following a commercial break, or I could walk onto set and take a seat once Trevor had introduced me. As I stroked the ears of my brand-new guide dog, Elton John, I knew that if I made the choice to walk out, it would have to be on my own. My millions of social media followers didn't yet know that just a few weeks prior, I had to unexpectedly give up my guide dog Ben Ben after just eight months. I was still in shock myself, still processing and coming to terms with the reality that I had just spent the last three weeks training with a new dog all over again. This interview with Trevor couldn't have come at a better time. After weeks of stress and tears, I was feeling numb and exhausted beyond belief, I needed something positive to hold on to and this felt like the opportunity of a lifetime. Getting to celebrate the thirty-second anniversary of the Americans with Disabilities Act on national television was the perfect distraction from the disastrous year I'd had.

Even though it would be risky, the decision was obvious to me. No matter what could happen, anything from falling flat on my face, or worse, getting disoriented navigating my way to the seat, I was going to walk out on my own. And I was going to make sure everyone saw me strut my stuff, sliding my cane across the floor with every step. My entire career—hell, nearly my entire life—has been devoted to moving the needle forward on authentic media representation of the disabled community, so there was no way I'd be passing up this moment to show every late-night viewer just how fabulous a blind girl could be!

While it may sound simple to most people, I knew that walk wouldn't be easy for me, but nothing in my life really has been or probably ever will be.

My therapist recently told me: "You're an extraordinary person. You've lived an extraordinary life, and that's something that everybody thinks they want. What many people don't understand is that to be extraordinary, you don't just get the extraordinarily amazing things, you also have to be the person who goes through the extraordinarily difficult ones. Most people wouldn't be willing to put up with the pain, hardships, and challenges you have, even if it means they'd get to enjoy an extraordinary life at the end. It doesn't matter how amazing your life looks to other people, you've had to weather a really harsh storm to get to live under the rainbow, and even now, it's still going to storm sometimes."

My social media feed, red carpet appearances, or global travels may appear to show a pretty pristine life, but behind the scenes, things have been far from glamorous. Though admittedly, that night on **The Daily Show** sure was one of the more glamorous ones. After a seven-minute interview that felt like ten seconds, I walked offstage only to be chased down by Trevor himself, who looked at me and said, "You need to be doing more... you need to write a book." So, Trevor, this one's for you.

INTRODUCTION

I used to tell people that I started speaking when I was five years old. After some confusion, I realized that people thought that meant I had spoken my first word at five years old, so now I clarify that I started PUBLIC speaking when I was five years old. Trust me, I spoke my first word, "banana," well before that age, and it's been a challenge to get me to shut my mouth ever since.

I know that five is rather young to first grace the stage with a microphone in hand, but my life has always been a little unusual, much like me. I was just six months old when my family began the journey to seeking a diagnosis for the concerning eye and head movements my grandfather noticed I was making while holding me in his arms. After many tests to rule out scary options like cancer, my parents were informed that I had spasmus nutans syndrome, a condition that typically occurs between six months to one year in age but goes away on its own within two years. It's characterized by rapid eye movements, head nodding, and a stiff neck position. Basically, I was like a little baby bobblehead, but not to worry, I was going to be fine! I don't know what the stats are now, but at the time, my parents were told it was a one-in-a-million diagnosis, so I often remind my parents that, for better or worse, they were blessed with a one-in-a-million daughter!

Unfortunately, this was far from the end of my medical journey, and I'd spend the next four years of my life going through exploratory tests and even surgeries to try to figure out what was going on. They say there's no use in crying over spilt milk, but when you're spilling it as much as I did, it's certainly cause for concern. They wanted to understand why I was so clingy at night in a way that was clearly more than a child's fear of the dark. Why I was walking into things, not yet reading or writing, and just generally acting differently from my peers and older brother. Eventually, the full diagnosis would come, and my parents were told it was a "dramatic" one, which I believe was foreshadowing for how dramatic I, and my life, would be.

One morning, just shy of my fifth birthday, the news came. My mom, Niamh, was out shopping to prepare for her upcoming trip home to Ireland to visit family, and my dad, Peter, was home looking after my brother, Brady, and me. Our cherry-red '90s home phone rang, and, not thinking much of it, my dad grabbed the receiver. He was expecting something quick, like a telemarketer trying to upsell him on cable, but instead he was greeted by the familiar French-Canadian voice of my doctor. In that moment, he received the diagnosis that would change all of our lives forever. Just two words: retinitis pigmentosa.[1] It was every parent's worst nightmare and the diagnosis mine had feared for years. I was going blind, and there was nothing anyone could do to stop it. Things were only going to get harder from here.

My mom arrived home with her arms filled with groceries, never expecting what my dad would tell her. They were in shock, unsure how to feel. In some strange twist of fate, later that very day my mom would pick up our local newspaper, and on the front cover was a little girl with her first white cane in hand. My mom knew in that moment that she could sink and pull me down with her, or she could swim and hold me up as she went. She chose to swim.

For my mom, swimming meant grabbing on to any floaty she could to hold her up when she felt too weak to keep kicking on her own. For her and my dad, this came in the form of activism. My parents didn't want to sit back and just watch me go blind, feeling helpless. They came across the Ending Blindness Foundation, which funded research to find a cure for RP and other blinding retinal diseases. They wanted to know that, whether it would make a difference or not, they were going to try to do something to change my future. This

---

1. If at any point while reading this book you find yourself saying, "Ableism? O&M? Vision itinerant? Huh, what's that?!" then I encourage you to look at the back of the book, where you'll find [my own personal] definitions for any disability- or blindness-related terms I use that may be confusing for the newbs.

meant putting a lot of time, effort, and energy into fundraising for Ending Blindness.

Like many charities, they were in need of a cute kid to pull at the heartstrings of donors (we'll discuss how problematic this is later on, don't worry) and asked my parents if I'd be willing to step onstage at their biggest fundraising event of the year—a motorcycle ride, of all things. All I had to do was wave the starting flag with a big smile on my face and say six simple words: "Ladies and gentlemen, start your engines!" And with that, the race, and my eventual public speaking career, were off to a start!

"Ahem, so now it's time to open up your hearts ... and your wallets." The audience laughed. From the moment my tiny hand wrapped around that microphone, I felt unstoppable. While most people may fill with fear when standing in front of an audience, I immediately felt more alive than ever before. My parents thought this was a onetime thing, but no, no, my friends, I had other plans. Some gossipy neighbors thought my parents forced me into all this charitable work as a kid, but it was quite the opposite. I BEGGED for them to let me do more, it was never enough. I spent the better half of the next decade speaking at all sorts of events. Whether it be a fancy dinner or a sweaty bicycle race, I was at a fundraiser and doing my thing, even if I had to stand on a chair to be seen above the podium. Over time my speaking increased from just that famous one-liner to three-, five-, or even ten-minute speeches that my dad would help me write until I was old enough to write them myself. I'd tirelessly memorize and practice them, performing each one to perfection with all the confidence of a theatre kid. I felt a deep longing for the stage.

But by fourteen, I had lost the majority of my vision much younger and faster than the doctors had predicted, and while the vision loss was unimaginably difficult, it was made ten times worse by ableism and how the rest of society treated me. I decided that the only way to avoid being hurt by the world was to avoid the world entirely and spend as much time as possible in the comfort and safety of my bedroom.

I stopped public speaking, I stopped performing, I stopped doing all of these different things that I was passionate about and that made me ... me. These things gave me life, they made me FEEL alive, but I didn't really want to be alive. I was suicidal. I just wanted to hide myself away from the world and pretend I didn't exist. I believed that if I hid myself away, the world couldn't hurt me anymore.

One night, I was at a fundraiser for Ending Blindness, this time not out of choice, but out of my parent's desperation to get me out of the house and back into an environment I once thrived in. I was bitter, I didn't want to be there. This thing that I had once loved so much now filled me with disgust because of the lies Ending Blindness and the doctors had sold my family and me.

"There'll be a cure within ten years of her diagnosis."

"There's a supplement you can get from Switzerland that will slow down the progression of your vision loss."

I believed their optimism because I was a child, and I thought that adults always told the truth. My parents believed them, because why wouldn't they trust the experts? Ending Blindness encouraged me: "All of your hard work and fundraising efforts will help us find a cure." But my vision was continuing to rapidly decline, and I was done trusting that life would ever get better than this dark emotional hellscape. I sat at the table, despondent, pushing my food around my plate with a fork. "Oh, I love your necklace!" my mom's voice called out to the woman on my right. Now that, that caught my attention. While I had no interest in discussing the latest research, I still had interest in discussing the latest trends. "What is it?" My face lit up with intrigue. The woman, a vision researcher, grabbed my hand and brought it to her neck. "H ... O ... P ... E." She traced out those four simple letters. "It's all we have." In silence, I took in those words. "Hope ... it's all we have." And I knew she was right. It was hope that I had lost and it was hope that I needed to find. Hope for better days, hope for healing, hope for a life that was more than I could currently envision. I wasn't sure how I'd get there but this was the start of my journey.

After about a year of intense therapy and some soul-searching, those words finally fully clicked. I was sitting in the doctor's office with my mom, cracked leather seat sticking to the undersides of my thighs in my light blue denim short shorts, when seemingly out of nowhere, I turned to her with a sense of urgency. "I have to start public speaking again." I knew I needed to find a way to make everything I had been through mean something. All the struggles couldn't be for nothing. There had to be greater purpose to my pain, and I knew that in order to find that purpose, I couldn't sit back and be angry that the world didn't understand me. All that was doing was keeping me down. I could choose to remain a victim, or I could choose to be a survivor, but to do that I would need to take an active role in changing the way society perceived me.

I knew how ignorant the world was when it came to blindness, or disability as a whole. I was facing it on a daily basis. From microaggressions to downright discrimination, I had seen it all (or should I say, I had "felt" it all, since apparently blind people aren't allowed to use words like "look" or "see"). But society wasn't going to begin to unlearn and relearn if someone wasn't willing to step up and teach them. I didn't quite know if I had it in me or, honestly, what it even meant at the time, but I knew I had to try, because the alternative—remaining in this state of wallowing in my circumstances—wasn't working. Somewhere deep down inside of me, I knew that I didn't want to live a life of bitterness and self-pity, and it was time to do something different. Every day I started telling myself, "If you don't change anything in your life, then nothing in your life is going to change." And I worked toward changing for the better.

I chose to stop being a passenger in my journey to recovery and start being the driver. I might not be able to drive a car, but I could still grab the steering wheel of my own life and take control again, navigating my way to where I want to go. Until this point, I had been going through the motions of recovery, guided by my parents and the team of professionals they had hired to support me. They had all gotten me to the point where I finally believed a different future was possible. I was strong enough to fight for myself and focus on rebuilding my life. The truth is, before I could change the way others saw me, I needed to change the way I saw myself.

I was learning that it was okay to grieve the loss of the girl I'd been, and the life I'd thought I was going to have. Grieving the death of yourself while trying to figure out how to keep living is a profound experience. Facing pain at that depth robbed me of my innocence. I was still young, but believe me, I was no longer a child. My youth had been stolen from me by years of trauma, bullying, and a deep sense of isolation, but it was time to surrender, to let that go while embracing and discovering my new, inescapable reality. I knew that I deserved to, and could, have a life that felt worth living again. But healing is never linear, and my journey would have a lot of unexpected twists and turns.

Along the way I'd eventually learn how to take back my power and finally speak up for myself. And in doing so, I've shared a lot of my life publicly but would you believe, there's even more I've kept hidden? These secrets aren't being held out of shame, I just honestly haven't known where to start untangling the messy web of emotional damage. It's taken me a long time to figure out how to open up about these past demons and even longer to extract meaning from them. I don't want my work to simply be an exploration of tragedy tourism. I want you to walk away feeling better off having read this book. So in the pages that follow there will be equal parts loss and resilience, the duality that is life. There will be some hard truths, but hopefully just as many important lessons. I want to bring you into my world: a world of feeling, and often being, unseen.

TIME TO GET TO WORK

Growing up knowing the statistics of unemployment within my community was pretty terrifying. At the time I was told that 80 percent of blind people were unemployed in Canada, where I grew up, and 70-80 percent in America, where I live now. This is something I had heard discussed around me my entire life, whether it be from my O&M or vision itinerant, life skills teacher, or my parents; I grew up knowing that my likelihood of finding employment was significantly lower due to my disability.

As a teenager, you hear about the importance of getting work experience and beginning to build up your résumé to set yourself up for success in the future. For me, this felt especially important. It felt like, more than anyone else, I had to prove myself, my worth, my value, and why I should be considered a desirable candidate for future employment. I didn't just have to check the boxes, I had to add new, bigger and better ones. Other people can just be "good enough," but I would have to be GREAT. Perfect isn't perfect enough when you're disabled, because ... no matter how perfect you are, the world will never view disability as perfect. The high standards I set for myself stemmed from fear. I was coping with the fear of my unknown future and the hardships I was almost sure to face by trying to be the best version of blindness anyone had ever seen. (Spoiler alert! It's impossible.)

When I began to dream up my new future as a blind woman, it was hard to imagine what jobs I could have. The world was quick to show and tell me all the things I wasn't capable of, so I wasn't foolish enough to think I could just walk into my local grocery store and apply to work the cash register or be a server at a restaurant like most teens around me. Finding a cash register with braille buttons or a screen reader probably wasn't going to happen, and I knew it would be pretty difficult to navigate carrying food from kitchen to table with just one hand while holding my guide dog's harness in the other. No, if I wanted to have a part-time job in high school like my peers, I'd have to think outside the box.

Given I had spent so much of my life volunteering, I understood all of the good that could come from it. I had been a youth ambassador for Ending Blindness and even planned my own fundraisers for them, like my fourteenth birthday donation drive, which I was told raised hundreds of thousands of dollars. In many ways, I knew volunteering was basically work experience, just without the paycheck. I'll be honest, though: as an avid beauty and fashion lover, I wanted a paycheck to fund my love of shopping, but I understood the uphill battle ahead of me to get one. I figured I could start by finding a local spot to volunteer with, show them how capable I was, and maybe, just maybe, it could turn into a paying gig someday.

After brainstorming my options for a bit but coming up short on ideas of jobs I actually thought I could do as a blind teenager, it finally came to me...summer camp! I grew up spending my summers in the sun, going from horseback riding and pottery, to acting and tennis camps, and loved every minute of it. I mean, I already knew all the lyrics to every campfire song ever written—it was perfect! So what better way to spend my summers now than volunteering at camps where I could help bring that same magic to other kids? About a five-minute drive down the road from my house was a big, beautiful, modern YMCA, with floor-to-ceiling windows, not one but two swimming pools, and countless activities. I had spent my childhood enjoying the space and figured it would be an easy starting point.

One Saturday afternoon, I walked in, application in hand. I approached the man behind the front desk, and we got to chatting. "I'm here to look into volunteering," I said with a smile on my face. He looked at me in confusion and asked, "Why aren't you applying for a job?" I had a list ready in my head of reasons why I didn't think I could be a counselor. I probably wouldn't be good at saving a drowning camper, and I certainly wouldn't be good with head counts or keeping visual track of the children. Would parents even trust me? He pointed out that there are ways of working around these things. "You should stop underestimating yourself and go for it." NEVER one to underestimate myself, I realized he was right and that's exactly what I was accidentally doing. And there was only one way to fix it. So that day, I scrapped my original plan and took a leap of faith.

Shortly after, I got the call to go in for my first job interview, and I was SO nervous. I put some flared yoga pants on and my nicest turquoise top with a silky cream belt tied around the waist.[2] I slid my feet into some black flats that I found at the back of my closet from my old private school uniform (I promise the outfit is even worse than you're picturing), and together, with my guide dog's harness in hand, Gypsy and I walked into the YMCA. It's mostly a blur (haha), but I remember answering some of the classic interview questions: strengths, weaknesses, blah, blah, blah. I can tell you that current Molly would answer "weaknesses" with "sight," but I'm fairly certain past Molly didn't quite have the confidence to make that joke yet, so I likely answered by saying that I tend to talk too much, which is ... still true. Despite this flaw, I was hired on the spot!

One thing I didn't expect was that this summer job would be so much more than singing "Boom Chicka Boom" and "The Great Big Moose" while trying not to burn my pale Irish skin. This job led to a year-round position as a rock-climbing instructor.

---

[2] Here's a random fact about me! I basically have a "photographic" memory of every outfit I've ever worn related to major events in my life. Some might say it's a useless skill, but look at it here, coming in handy!

YES, you read that right: at the end of the summer, my boss offered me the opportunity to work in the YMCA's rock-climbing gym, which would include running a group class for children ages five to ten on Sunday mornings and belaying anyone else who wanted to climb. This meant I'd be in charge of harnessing people up and keeping them safe on the other end of the rope as they climbed. I should probably mention that, aside from being blind, I was also only four ten and a half (yes, the half matters) and about eighty-five pounds. I was basically the same size as the ten-year-olds. I know—what could go wrong?

As you can imagine, I had some initial concerns. What if parents didn't want to put the life of their child in the hands of someone who was not only the same size as most of them, but who couldn't even see them? Bringing these concerns to my new boss, I wasn't too sure how he'd react, but I could hear the smile in his voice when he assured me, "If these parents don't want a fully qualified and trained instructor to belay their kids—regardless of your blindness—then they can take their children to climb somewhere else." This simple statement showed his belief in me, and that's the exact kind of encouragement I needed. If he believed in me, maybe I could try to believe in me too.

Pity is something a lot of people are quick to dole out to disabled people, which (at the risk of speaking for an entire, very diverse community) is NEVER what we are looking for. I don't want people to feel bad for me; I want them to have empathy. So often we are either put on a pedestal and praised for simply existing, or we are looked down upon with sadness. We are used as a source of hope and inspiration, or looked at with those **I guess my life could be worse** eyes. I'm told I'm "so brave" and "courageous" when I'm just grabbing my morning cup of coffee, or they so bluntly say, "I could never do what you do. If I went blind, I'd kill myself." People dehumanize us, and we are othered from society, thought of as less than or separate from, instead of people realizing that we are YOU. And someday, YOU could be us. Most disabilities are acquired due to age, accident, or illness. We are the only minority community that anyone can join at any time. We as disabled people are frequently discriminated against, but disability itself does not discriminate. It doesn't matter what color your skin is, your religious beliefs, who you vote for, or what naturopathic supplements you take. You and your loved ones may one day be disabled, and the reality is, if you live long enough, you will be in some capacity. And being disabled doesn't change who you are, it changes how you live. We want the same things out of life as you, we just function in slightly different ways, which, realistically, disabled or not, everyone does.

 When my boss assured me with those words, it showed that he thought of me as equal and deserving. Not deserving out of the "goodness of his heart," not deserving out of a charitable duty, but out of respect and a willingness to build understanding for what he might not understand. He had an open mind that actually helped expand my own. He wouldn't be willing to lose business just to give me a chance—he thought I could do it, and now, so did I.

On Sunday morning, I headed into work, and as I was completing the figure-eight knot for a first-time climber, her mom approached me: "Who's that cute dog over there?"

As I continued to feed the rope through my grigri, I absentmindedly replied, "That's my guide dog." And immediately, I regretted my decision. I could feel the discomfort radiating off of her. It was silent for a moment, and then I wished it was.

She began loudly insisting that one of my coworkers take over for me because "HOW is a blind girl supposed to keep my daughter safe?" In that moment, my stomach dropped, and my mouth dried up. I felt like if I tried to speak, I would just trip over my words, or worse, burst into tears. Shocked, embarrassed, and ashamed, I started thinking, **Maybe she's right. Maybe I shouldn't be here**. Self-doubt raced through me. I felt less than, a feeling that's sadly all too familiar to a disabled person.

Her words stung like those of my bullies. With that brief encounter, years of feeling inadequate and all of the internalized ableism I'd been fighting deep inside began to bubble to the surface. But then, I heard the words of my boss replay in my mind, and I knew he wouldn't put up with this. His belief in me gave me the strength to believe in myself, even if only for a fleeting moment. I looked at her and, as calmly as possible, voice quivering, I said, "I'm just as qualified and capable of belaying your daughter as anyone else who works in this gym. Unfortunately, my coworkers aren't available, but I'm more than happy to belay her. I promise she'll be safe with me. I do this multiple times a week and have never had an accident or issue, but if you don't feel comfortable, you can take her elsewhere." And just like that, she sat back on the bench and watched her child climb happily with me for the next half hour.

My first working experiences at summer camp were positive thanks to a supportive boss who made me feel like the ways I could contribute were greater than what I lacked. In fact, following my first summer at camp I received a major award for the mentorship I provided the campers in foster care. But sadly, for so many in my community, their work experiences would look a lot more like my experiences thereafter.

One warm spring evening I was hanging out with some of my camp friends who I'd worked with in previous summers. We had begun discussing our excitement for the upcoming camp season when my usually loudmouthed friend, Katie, started to get quiet. She was a few years older than me and had a new position. She was finally in a leadership role, something she was very deserving of. This gave her access to the hiring room, where she, along with a committee of other staff, discussed who to hire and who to fire, but we all knew better than to ask her about that side of things.

While I hadn't received news yet that I was invited back to work at camp again, I figured it was coming soon. None of my work friends aside from Katie had heard yet either, so I wasn't concerned. I was well liked, had had a successful few years in the same position, and didn't think much of it. I mean, why wouldn't I be hired again?

Katie started to seem a bit uncomfortable but managed to stammer out, "Um... there is something I feel like I should tell you, Molls. I don't really know how to say this, but... when your application came across the desk, the new camp director immediately said she didn't see why we should bother hiring you and said in a super-dismissive tone that you can just volunteer."

I immediately felt my cheeks get hot, flushing with emotion. **This woman hasn't even met me yet; how can she even begin to make a judgment on whether or not I can do this job? Besides, my résumé is proof that I can! How am I supposed to react to this news? What am I supposed to say?**

Thankfully, I didn't have to say anything; Katie could see it on my face. "We all fought for you! Everyone in that room told her they'd quit if she didn't hire you again. We told her that you are the definition of what camp is all about and it wouldn't be the same without you. So many other staff and campers would be disappointed if you weren't there."

As kind and heartwarming as it was to know that my coworkers felt so passionately about my right to work alongside them, it was truly heartbreaking to hear that my new boss had such a stark difference in her view of me from my previous boss. It was like having all your own inner demons, your own dark, mean thoughts, echoed back to you. Those same feelings of insecurity, inadequacy, and even anger once again felt like they were right at the surface, wanting to break free. But I instead just put on a brave face, smiled, and pretended I was fine. "Thanks, Katie, you're the best." I acted like the discrimination was nothing new... because it wasn't.

When the position was officially offered to me just one week later, I took it. Unfortunately, it was short-lived. Unsurprisingly, my new boss treated me terribly. She and a few of the other new camp staff clearly made it their mission to make my life as difficult as possible. Classic mean-girl energy... There were cutting remarks and backhanded comments, not to mention they would never give me opportunities to contribute and sometimes just straight-up acted like I wasn't there. They gave me the impression that they wanted me to quit, and I'm sad to say that I gave in.

"You have to pick your battles" is a line I've heard from my parents a few too many times. Being blind, the battles can happen almost daily. If I fight every little obstacle in front of me, I'll spend my time exhausted, angry, and in a perpetual state of negativity. As much as I wanted to be the girl who stood up for EVERY injustice she saw...I didn't have it in me quite yet. This felt like a battle I would never win, and I didn't feel like trying to convince someone of my worth when they didn't want to see it, so I moved on instead.

There's a world in which I could have experienced this prejudice the moment I walked into my first job interview or following my first summer of work. This kind of attitude or mindset is the reality that a lot of disabled people face. You fight for the right to be there, and then you're made to feel so unwanted that you eventually burn out and leave. Up to one in four people living in the United States today have some form of a disability, and the vast majority, about 80 percent, are unemployed. Globally, over a billion people are disabled. We are a large community that isn't going anywhere, and not working with us is a major missed opportunity.[3] And you and I both know it would be a damn shame to miss out on having my adorable guide dog as your coworker.

I can confidently say that I bring a lot of positive qualities to the table (and he brings a lot of paw-sitive ones as well), as do many of my disabled peers, but what we offer seems to be so easily overlooked. People fixate on what they assume we can't do. But just because you imagine **you** wouldn't be able to do something without your left arm, with reduced hearing, or with

---

[3]. Check out the CDC and the World Health Organization websites for more fun statistics!

your eyes closed, doesn't mean we can't. We live these lives every day, and our experience of doing something with our disability day in and day out is very different from you trying to do it once.

I'm grateful for my first boss because without him, I might have given up hope. But in a weird way, I'm equally as grateful for my second boss because she gave me a reality check and prepared me for my likely future. That negative workplace experience was the first like it for me, but not the last, and it is reflective of the reality of life for many disabled people seeking employment. As messed up as it sounds, it almost feels like a rite of passage to being a disabled person in the workforce.

As I continued seeking work opportunities in my late teens and early twenties, I had a number of similar experiences where I was denied a job specifically because I'm blind. This even includes an UNPAID volunteer role at a leadership conference. The reason they didn't want me there? Because I couldn't do very important leadership duties like writing the name tags for the participants. There was also another summer camp that, after verbally promising me a job for the next camp season, did not employ me because, "We'd have to give you a co-counselor, and we can't afford to do that. Hiring two of you to do the job for one just doesn't make financial sense." And sure, I'd believe that load of BS, IF they didn't already have plenty of groups at their camp that required two counselors to work together.

How many times can you put yourself out there, only to face rejection after rejection based on a core part of who you are?

In our community, having a job is a privilege, and we know that, which makes it really hard for many of us to stand up for ourselves or our rights. Like any toxic or abusive relationship, you can find yourself feeling trapped in a situation that isn't healthy, but you're grateful to have a job, ANY JOB, so you're willing to put up with less-than-fair treatment just to have the opportunity pay your bills. With negative experiences like these, especially if you don't have any positive ones to balance it out, it would be very easy to feel discouraged, hopeless, or want to give up on even trying to find a fulfilling job. We need employers to be educated and aware, so they feel more confident and empowered to give us the same opportunities as non-disabled people.

BUT DAD, I DON'T WANNA GO TO COLLEGE

My eighteenth birthday fell halfway through my senior year of high school.[4] Like most seniors, I was deep in the midst of trying to figure out what my next plans were... What the hell am I going to do with the rest of my life? I was touring universities and looking at courses, but nothing felt quite right, and frankly, I was SO done with school.

Throughout my childhood, I switched schools five times in an attempt to find the best support and accommodations for me as a student who was progressively going blind. Given that the traditional school system is built on visual learning, and shockingly, I'm NOT a visual learner, it was difficult to say the least. Couple that with vision and needs that are constantly changing and having trouble socially, continuing to expose myself to this unique form of torture while acquiring student loan debt didn't exactly sound alluring. Nothing about any

---

4. I'm an Aquarius, for those who might be wondering. And I'm sure if you know anything about astrology, this is not surprising in the slightest.

of these university degrees I was looking at held any appeal. "I just want to graduate and get straight to work," I kept telling my parents, not caring how unrealistic this was. The only thing I felt passionate enough about to consider pursuing as a career was motivational speaking, and there isn't exactly a degree that aligns with that. I felt like if I was really going to make it in the industry, it was best to get straight to it and not waste any more time. Eighteen-year-old me was not playing around.

For my birthday that year, I got tickets to see a speaker who was the founder of Evolving as One, a very large and successful social enterprise (a business that intends to do good with the money they make). I'll admit, I actually hadn't heard of the guy or his company, BUT a good family friend knew how much I loved public speaking and philanthropy, so when they heard he was coming to town they got me two tickets. Richard (who went by Dick) ran an organization with both local and global initiatives to help empower youth and give them access to necessary resources. Evolving as One (EAO for short) offered things ranging from sustainable clothing and accessories, to youth volunteer trips to the countries it served. They even had books and speakers and ran massive events in stadiums around the world with A-list celebrities gracing the stage to promote their noble causes.

After receiving the tickets and looking into his work, I couldn't wait to see Dick speak. He was someone who had made such a difference in the world by sharing his story, inspiring and empowering people the very way I wanted to. He was traveling the world, speaking on big stages to thousands of people, uplifting, motivating, educating, and sparking important conversations that needed to be had. I guess in many ways, I had been doing something similar, just on a very small scale. He was positively affecting the masses with his words and his work... That was the type of change I could only dream of achieving. **How amazing would it be to live a life with so much impact?** I thought to myself.

On a cold, snowy winter evening, I bundled up in my warmest coat and boots, with Gypsy and my mom, to head to the event. We raced into the theatre to get the best seats possible—not for me, I can't see a damn thing regardless of where I sit, but Gypsy was a long-legged gal (the only tall one in our family), and it was important to find a spot that would be convenient and comfortable for everyone. Typically, the front row is best because it gives her ample room to lie down, while also not getting in anyone's way. The seats weren't preassigned; it was first come, first served, and we were determined to be first!

We managed to stumble upon two empty seats in the front row on the far-left side of the stage. For forty-five minutes, Dick shared stories from his life that left me in awe. You could certainly say I lived, laughed, loved it. I felt elated, more sure than ever that THIS was my future.

After the applause died down, he spent fifteen minutes taking questions from the audience. I desperately wanted to ask him something, but felt far too nervous to raise my hand up. My mom could tell I was waffling back and forth, so when he announced that he had time for one more question, she loudly whispered in my ear, "He can't see it!" as she grabbed my wrist, lifting it into the air for me. "Let's go with you: right there in the front row!" he said loudly, and then to my surprise, my mom leaned over. "That's you!" She knew that without her telling me, I'd have no idea that I was the chosen one.

Now that I had my big moment, as clearly and confidently as I could, I shared, "I'm in grade twelve, and I'm trying to figure out where to go to school next year, but nothing feels quite right. I want to be a motivational speaker. Do you have any recommendations of courses I could take for that?"

He followed this up with some flowery, generic answer about the importance of following your dreams, which wasn't exactly helpful in that moment. I wanted specifics; I wanted a road map to follow so that I could be where he was one day. He was selfless, living his life to help make the lives of others better... How could I not want that? Thankfully, after wrapping up his less-than-satisfying answer, he ran offstage and came directly over to me. A crowd began to form around us of people wanting autographs and photos with Dick. He quickly handed me a business card and said, "Reach out to my assistant." A little confused, I didn't quite know what this meant, or where it would lead, but I was intrigued and ready to find out.

Sitting down at my computer the next day, I prepared to type out an email where I reiterated my question from the night before and attached my résumé so they could get an idea of my history and experience. I was hoping it would allow them to better recommend the best next steps for me. After hitting send, I opened my email every day, eagerly searching for a reply, only to be disappointed once again... no response. I told myself that this was to be expected. I mean, why would they even bother? They had bigger things to deal with, like solving world hunger (literally).

After what felt like months of waiting with anticipation (but was probably no more than two weeks), I finally heard back from someone at EAO who essentially said, "You can't apply to be a speaker here; we don't accept applications." Hmm... not exactly what I was hoping for. I'm not sure where the miscommunication happened, but clearly somewhere along the line, wires were crossed. **Since when was I applying for a job?** I thought to myself. I just wanted a little advice! Looking back, maybe this is the first red flag I missed... their email showed a lack of care and basic kindness, not to mention overlooking simple details. We certainly weren't starting out on the right foot.

Feeling dismissed, I knew I couldn't just sit back and expect a new opportunity to fall into my lap, so I continued to pursue other alternatives, including looking at yet another university. It was a small school not too far from home but far enough away that I'd have a bit more freedom, which I desperately craved, even if it did scare me a little. I'm sure most eighteen-year-olds can relate to the feeling of wanting to start to break away from family life and begin to become your own adult self. But, being disabled, the need and want for greater independence is on an entirely different level.

I know that I'll never achieve the same autonomy that sighted people have, if only because I can't do basic things like drive a car or go for a run or bike ride without help. My lack of independence at times isn't necessarily because I'm incapable but rather because my body or the world around me doesn't allow for it. Due to this, I often spend my time striving for the most freedom and independence that's possible with the limitations I face. I wish I could say that I can do anything and everything, but the reality is that unless and until the world is more accessible and accommodating to disabled people, that's not possible. And it's a realization that comes with a lot of heavy emotions... self-pity, sadness, anger, resentment, feeling unworthy, not good enough, less valuable, the list goes on. But these feelings aren't helpful, so while I let myself feel them sometimes because they can be unavoidable, I don't let myself live with this victim mentality. And while I can't do anything and everything the way I wish I could or the way that others can, I'll still figure out a work-around to get the task at hand done... even if it means calling in some backup!

My good friend Mark, from my YMCA camp days, was currently in his second year at this very school, so I reached out, and he suggested he give me a one-on-one tour. **You mean, I can avoid the crowds of group tours and get to catch up with a great friend? Sign me up.**

After a day of exploring the campus and all it had to offer alongside Gypsy, my mom, and Mark, my interest was admittedly a little piqued. I wasn't completely sold, but it was the most sold on college I had been up until this point. It felt safe... a small school, close enough to home but still far enough away. It was a good school with a solid reputation, had some courses that aligned with my interests in social justice, and I heard some decently positive feedback about their disability support program from other blind people I knew who had studied there. Plus, the fact that I already had a friend there was a huge bonus! This MIGHT actually be an option.

On the car ride home, I discussed this with my mom while texting my friend Brooke from school about how badly I needed my nails done (because... priorities), and she suggested we meet up and get them done together. My mom rerouted the car to drop me off at the nail salon. As we pulled up, I noticed that I had a voicemail. Because everyone important to me knows to text me instead of calling (I am a millennial, after all!), I was unsure as to what call I could have missed.

Standing outside the salon, phone pressed against my ear, I heard a singsongy voice on the other end that sounded slightly embarrassed but very optimistic. In a friendly and enthusiastic tone, she explained, "I'm Sharon, and I'm the head of the speakers bureau at Evolving as One." As the voicemail continued, I learned that my résumé had somehow landed upon her desk, and while her assistant had disregarded me in his prior email, her energy couldn't have been more different. Full of compliments, she warmly invited me to the office. "I'd love to chat and get to know you a little better and hear about your goals and future plans."

My jaw dropped. I looked over, wide-eyed, at Brooke as she stood beside me and then toward my mom's car, which I could still hear idling nearby. Surprised and hopeful, I eagerly shared the contents of the message, not quite knowing what to do next.

What ensued in the coming weeks was a flurry of emails, phone calls, and car rides to Toronto, where I found myself sitting in a modern office surrounded by glass walls, taking meetings my eighteen-year-old self did not quite feel equipped to handle. After sitting down with Sharon for an hour, she informed me that Dick, the founder of EAO, wanted to have a formal meeting.

Me? He wants to meet little old me? He spent his days rubbing shoulders with the rich and famous. What could he possibly want to meet with me for? It was hard to process it.

My parents and I made sure to show up well before the meeting was scheduled to begin. "If you're not early, you're late!" my dad told me. "Busy men like him are running from one meeting to another, if you're not there when he shows up, he's moving on!" We pulled into the parking lot of the Starbucks Dick had selected for our meeting. I was filled with anticipation.

Sitting on the hard wooden chair, I was looking like a little fangirl in my EAO chocolate-brown T-shirt with **YOU CAN CREATE CHANGE** emblazoned across the chest. When he did show up, he rushed in late with an air of importance around him and sat down at the table with us. A little starstruck, I didn't even have a chance to say hi before he launched into what I now know was a job interview. All business. Straight to the point. As if he were firing a gun, he hurled hard-hitting questions at me, and as they hit me like bullets, I tried my best to give the most impressive answers possible. "Who are you and why should I care? Give me your thirty-second elevator pitch." **An elevator pitch? What is that?** I thought to myself, before launching into some semblance of an answer. My years of improv training and acting classes really came in handy, and I managed to keep my composure as he looked around the table at my parents and announced to me with the utmost bravado, "I'd like you to move into the city and start touring as a full-time speaker. We'll get you an apartment and an assistant and give you media training. Starting in September, I want you on stages in stadiums around North America."

I was almost too stunned to speak. Somehow I managed to stammer out, "But...but I still have six more months of school before I graduate."

"That won't work," he interjected. "I need you to start touring when our next event kicks off in September. I'm very connected with the school board; I'll make sure you graduate on time." Not entirely sure what he meant by that, I nodded while he told us that he'd give us a few days to consider but he'd like an answer by the end of the week.

THIS IS WHAT DREAMS ARE MADE OF

While my peers were touring university dorm rooms, I was busy touring apartments in downtown Toronto, trying to decide whether I should live with a roommate or live alone, and asking myself questions like, "How close to the office is too close?" I ended up settling on living alone so that I wouldn't have to deal with reminding a roommate to put their shoes away when they took them off because I'd trip over them when I walked in the door. And to please not move my kombucha from one shelf to another in the fridge, because if you do, it's simply lost to me. My parents, who had lived with me for eighteen years, still made these mistakes, so I didn't really trust a perfect stranger to catch on or even care to. As a social person who'd always lived with other people (my family), I was a little fearful of the idea of going home every day to an empty apartment, but I knew Gypsy and I would manage to turn it into a cozy escape. The pros would outweigh the cons.

Conveniently enough, EAO owned a handful of properties surrounding the offices, and many of their young employees fresh out of university were living in the "staff housing." They presented me with the same deal they offered to everyone else on payroll: in exchange for taking a lower salary, they would provide my housing for free. They had a few empty units for me to pick from, and given that I obviously couldn't drive, commuting wasn't an option. And I knew that even if I took the full salary it wouldn't begin to cover the average cost of rent in Toronto. So I ended up going with one of their two-bed, one-bath units with a large patio and slanted ceiling. It was located on the same block as the office. And though I was concerned living that close would leave me with little to no separation between work and life, it was the safest option. Not having to cross any streets in rush-hour traffic to get to and from work? A blind girl's dream! Although this did mean I had no excuses for being late . . . I couldn't exactly claim there was bad traffic on my twenty-step commute.

It may have been spacious, but my new apartment left much to be desired. It had big windows with ample natural lighting, but the kitchen and bathroom were old and unrenovated. There was cheap, mismatched furniture throughout. **Oh well, beggars can't be choosers.** I sure wasn't going to complain. Besides, I've always loved interior makeovers, and now I had an entire apartment to transform! I could find a way to make this space totally my style, though it would have to be on a budget. Because after my housing was deducted from my pay, I was only making $20,000 a year (which, in 2012, was just about minimum wage given a forty-hour workweek). But hey, I was just happy to be able to graduate high school six months earlier than expected and have a good reason to skip out on university. Dick had indeed pulled some strings, and somehow I was able to get all the credits I needed to get my high school diploma early. And just like that, I was free and couldn't be happier about it. To think of the power this man had to pull something like that off...

In my senior year, I chose not to get a yearbook or pose for a graduation photo in a cap and gown. I didn't even go to my graduation. In fact, they had to call my parents to ask them to come pick up my diploma at the office. By the time grade twelve had rolled around, I'd viewed school as a necessary evil that I simply had to grin and bear until it was over. I saw it as a stepping stone that I had to walk across to get to where I wanted to go in life, and I was finally getting there. I held no emotional attachment to school or the idea of graduating, and none of these "milestones" felt important for me to partake in. Even now, I have no regrets. While those may be special memories for some, my school memories are mostly ones I wish I didn't have, and no yearbook photo or graduation walk would change that. (I don't know many blind people who would flip through their yearbook anyway.)

My dad and older brother were a little apprehensive at first because they're big believers in the traditional education system, but somehow, my free-spirited mom and I managed to convince them that skipping out on university wouldn't ruin all future opportunities for me. "School will always be there. I can go back and get a degree at some point in the future!" I suggested, while emotionally pleading my case. "This opportunity is once in a lifetime. It's a dream job for me. I don't care that the pay is low and the housing isn't anything to brag about!" Honestly, I felt like I had won the lottery. I could be PAYING money to learn at school, or I could be getting paid to learn in the real world. It felt like a no-brainer.

Dick had been able to deliver on everything he promised. From helping me graduate early so I could start touring, to the apartment in the city, so far, he'd been a man of his word. This also meant I got the assistant he'd mentioned. With all this change in my life, it was a lot of newness to take in. Thankfully, my assistant wasn't new to me. In my final two years of high school, I had a vision itinerant named Rebecca. She was beautiful: tall, with wavy bleach-blond hair and a sparkling smile to match her bubbly personality. She was ten years older than me and like the cool big sister I never had. Outside of school, we'd attend hot yoga classes on the weekends and even went to get tattoos together the summer before my senior year. When she found out about my big opportunity and that I'd require an assistant, she applied for a one-year leave of absence from the school board to come along with me. She would also opt into staff housing and would live alone in the unit below mine. We were the only two living in this big Victorian building. Well, I guess that's not exactly true. There was Gypsy, of course, and we would come to find a slew of unwanted furry guests...

On my very first night living alone in the big city I invited my friend Brooke to come sleep over in my guest room. After having dinner and drinks at the British pub around the corner, we decided to sit out and enjoy the end-of-summer sunset on my fourth-floor patio. As we listened to music and chatted about the future, she suddenly leaned over and pressed pause. "SHHH!" She fell silent.

Through nervous laughter, I asked, "What the hell is wrong with you?" I can confidently say that I was completely unprepared for what she was about to tell me.

"Don't freak out, but we're not alone up here."

"Um, excuse me?" (NOT the right thing to tell my true-crime-loving self on my FIRST night there.) With a shaky voice I whispered, "What the hell are you talking about?"

She paused and, without moving a muscle, she muttered, "There's an entire family of racoons up here, and the mama is NOT pleased that we're crashing her party." Claws in the air, Mama hissed as her four babies glared from behind. Gypsy, forever the optimist, thought she could likely reduce the tension and make a new furry friend in the process, so she started to inch toward her. Mama started circling, like a shark sussing out its prey. Brooke let out a loud shriek, jumping on top of her seat. "Oh my god, Molly. Stand on your chair."

In a panic, I yelled, "RESTER!" at Gypsy (the French command for "stay"). We quickly constructed a game plan.

This space was an entirely new environment for me, so I wasn't fully confident in navigating my way around yet. Somehow my patio felt too big and too small at the same time. With Mama closing in, it suddenly felt smaller than a New York City closet. And yet the five or six feet we had to go to get back inside felt as long as an Olympic-sized pool. We had to walk up three steps and open not one, but two doors to get inside, AND with Mama nearby... Mission Impossible. Brooke decided it was best to get Gypsy inside first, since she would likely be the first victim. While Mama was at the far side of the table, Brooke jumped down, grabbed Gypsy's collar, and ran. Throwing open the screen door, and then the heavy wooden one, she practically shoved Gypsy inside.

Oh god. Now it was just me, still standing on my chair, racoon still looming and Brooke looking at me wide-eyed from the other side of the screen. She knew I wouldn't be able to make it back inside without her help, so she once again waited for her moment. As I cowered in fear, she dashed out. "Jump and run!" she urged me, grabbing my wrist and pulling me along behind her. With adrenaline coursing through my veins, I leapt to the top of the stairs and dove through the door to safety. Not exactly the friendly neighbors I was hoping for. Thankfully, they soon left. And if you're reading this thinking I was being dramatic, then why don't you try evading wild raccoons with your eyes closed?

I wasn't going to let this little hiccup bring me down. Bright and early on Monday morning, I awoke with three hours to get myself ready to head into the office and begin my first real big-girl job. I blended up a smoothie, walked my guide dog, made my bed, brushed my teeth and hair, threw on some makeup and a pair of high heels. Instead of spending the last few weeks of summer going back-to-school shopping, I had gone off-to-work shopping. This included buying all the grown-up things like blazers, dress pants, heels, and red lipstick. I knew I had to find a way to make my acne-covered baby face and tiny frame look like I deserved to be sitting at a desk in a corporate office writing a speech I'd soon be delivering to twenty thousand people.

It wasn't long before the cracks began to appear in the shiny exterior of my new career. Going into the office when you have nothing to actually do at an office desk felt strange. I had been told by a prior speaker that he did not have to go in to work every day, he could write and practice his speeches at home, go in to rehearse, and focus his energy on touring. This rule had since changed, given his failure to succeed at EAO, and I was now made to go into the office for what felt like no other reason than to keep tabs on me and micromanage. For the most part, I just watched episodes of **Dr. Phil**[5] on YouTube with my laptop screen pointed at the wall behind me.

It was two weeks into my new job when I was hauled into a boardroom to rehearse my new speech for Dick. While he let me mostly write it myself, he basically told me what he wanted me to say (whether it was true or... only half-true) and was also instructing me on exactly how he wanted me to say it. He was my drill sergeant, and I was his faithful soldier, doing as I was told. After the longest hour, listening to his booming voice reaching a volume unnecessary for such a small room, "PAUSE, ONE, TWO, THREE, THEN YOU RAISE YOUR RIGHT HAND!" I walked out of the third-floor office, and as I approached the second floor, a kind coworker I had yet to meet stopped me on the stairs with concern in her voice. "Are you okay? We could all hear him from the floor below..."

"Oh yeah, don't worry about it! That's just Dick being Dick!" I said with one of those **if you know, you know** expressions on my face (I might have only been two weeks in, but I was already catching the vibes of my new working environment). Thankfully, I had grown thick skin from years of being bullied and had learned the art of people-pleasing. I could shut up and be exactly who he needed me to be, all with a smile on my face.

---

5. It was my guilty pleasure, ok?! We all have one.

UNSEEN

Just three weeks after walking into my first day on the job, I was already doing my sound check at a stadium in downtown Toronto, preparing to make my first appearance as the newest speaker for EAO. I had been to this very stadium countless times over the years, first to see Taylor Swift live in concert, and then to see her again. Next came Ed Sheeran, then Katy Perry, and then came... me? This couldn't be real. I stood backstage having a mic pack attached to the back of my leggings, cord snaking its way up the inside of my shirt, which was covered in gold-foiled branding from EAO, and a headset hooked behind my ears. A man taped a tiny mic to the side of my cheek. "There! That'll hold it in place!" he said, as I pinched myself. In less than twenty-four hours I'd be standing on that stage in front of twenty thousand middle and high school students, telling a story I wasn't quite sure I was ready to share. But Dick was ready for me to, so, ready or not, I was going to do it. All in the name of promoting EAO's newest campaign.

With my hair loosely curled by Rebecca, skinny jeggings on (listen, it was the look back then, okay?!), black slip-on Toms on my feet, and yet another XXS branded T-shirt from EAO, I was ready to take to the stage. Well, after the makeup artist helped cover up the breakout on my chin... THEN I'd be ready. My parents, brother, and even my grandparents, who had flown in from Ireland, stood in the stands next to Sharon. With Gypsy by my side, I fiddled nervously with the white-gold claddagh ring that's been living on my finger since my fifteenth birthday. I quickly muttered the words to my speech under my breath... I had been practicing for a week straight. I had every word, every movement, and every inflection down to a fine art, which Dick had carefully crafted for me.

Rebecca gave me a sighted guide up the stairs behind the stage and placed me on my mark. Then she brought Gypsy over to her mark too. It wasn't just me performing; Gypsy also had a vital role to play. I heard the hosts of the event say my name, and as cheering began, I started to count out my steps as I walked alone onto the T-shaped stage. **Eleven steps forward.** All my nerves disappeared. **Turn left. One, two, three, four. It starts to feel like an out-of-body experience. Five more steps and I hit my mark.** I took a moment to soak in the bright spotlights as they illuminated my face. All of my preparation, sleepless nights thinking through every mistake I could make, but when those lights hit me, a sense of peace washed away every doubt. You're laser focused. Nothing else exists. You don't have to think anymore, you just do. The idea of performing for that many people is so intimidating, you could never imagine that they would cease to exist, but I was so locked in with a mechanical precision. "One person..." I heard Martin Sheen's voice replaying in my head. Standing in the greenroom just moments earlier, between loving pets to

Gypsy he had mentored me with these words: "You're speaking to one person in that audience. Decide who it is and speak directly to them; forget everyone else exists." So that's exactly what I did. **You're speaking to the younger you**, I told myself; then I opened my mouth and the words began to flow out of me. And just like that, I hit every single line and used every single hand gesture that Dick had choreographed for this very moment, like a good little marionette doll.

A MOMENT OF SILENCE

"The world is a noisy place, and silence makes people feel uncomfortable. We fill our lives with chatter by leaving TVs on, blasting radios, headphones permanently attached to our ears, a constant stream of noise."

The campaign I was promoting was called **Be Silent**. The goal was to encourage the youth in attendance to take a vow of silence for twenty-four hours to raise awareness for voiceless communities. Of course, the most effective way for me to do this was to utilize my uniqueness, so that's exactly what I did.

A girl like me wouldn't have this opportunity if I wasn't willing to continue to package up my story in a pretty little box that I could hand out like candy for other people's enjoyment. In my experience, philanthropists often use pain and heartbreak to propel their message and increase engagement and donations. An ethical dilemma: Is it okay to exploit the trauma of a marginalized and oppressed person if they are willing and you are doing so to ultimately create a positive impact on said community? This is something I had unknowingly fallen victim to from such a young age... by eighteen, I still didn't know any better. I had been doing it in one way or another for organizations like Ending Blindness since I was five. I was the perfect prey, a natural oversharer who loved to talk to just about anyone and sought deep connections through storytelling and finding common bonds with strangers. Seemingly confident, extroverted, with a flair for the dramatics, I made for the ideal candidate to get this very specific job done. I was vulnerable, looking to please, and felt genuinely overwhelmed by how many problems in the world I wanted to help fix. I had always thought of charities as trustworthy, so trust I did.

"Now is the time to become aware of that uncomfortable silence again. Now is our time to be silent to give us the power to think. To give us the power to act. It is our time to stand up for what we believe in, to make the world a better place. I found my voice when I stood up against bullying. This is my story; this is why I am choosing to be silent."

To this day, I still don't really think the connection between speaking up AND going silent makes a whole lot of sense, but hey, Dick thought it did, and I was just there to play a part. I wasn't going to say a damn thing about it because I wasn't willing to risk upsetting him and losing this opportunity to make my dreams a reality. If I had to open up old wounds to make my boss happy, so be it. Besides, between the years of therapy and my brain's natural trauma response of dissociating, it basically felt like it was someone else's story by this point. I had managed to compartmentalize and separate myself from the darkness of my past and could recite it like I was reading lines from a fictional script. It just so happened that the fictional script was actually my real life.

"I want to tell you about a time when I was fourteen. I had an injured ankle and was at school on crutches. I had already spent the entire year as a target for bullies for being the girl that stood up for what she believed in." I mean, this isn't exactly why I was being bullied, but it fit the narrative, so for this moment, I went with it and continued on, "They made it their daily goal to make my life miserable. One day, a classmate asked me if I wanted to go for a walk with the popular girls. They actually wanted to hang out with me!" It wasn't exactly the "popular girls"; it was my old friends. Again, there's a lot more to this story, but I was only given five and a half minutes onstage, and it had been DRILLED into me that if I went over, even by just thirty seconds, the delay would ruin the rest of the show. So I made the story as concise as I could to allow for the showstopping moment that would soon occur.

"I knew they were bullies, but as I so desperately wanted friends, I agreed. We were walking down a huge hill. The grass at the bottom of the hill started to become uneven with roots. Branches started hitting me in the face. We ended up in a forest. I sat down and laid my crutches by my side. The next thing I heard was the sound of laughter, then the sound of my crutches being smashed against a tree. I knew they were broken. Then [pause for effect] I tried to stand up, and reach out for something to hold on to, but as soon as I put weight on my ankle, I collapsed face down onto the grass." When we worked on this portion of the speech, I remember being told something along the lines of, "Life isn't black and white; there's a lot of gray area in between. Sometimes adding a little drama to make the story more impactful is okay." It made me a bit uncomfortable, but Dick was the successful one, not me, so surely he knew what he was talking about, right? I was just lucky to be learning from the best, so with all the showmanship I could muster, I went on.

"My chest tightened, and I felt a lump grow in my throat. My eyes filled with tears, and as they started to pour down my cheeks, I wiped them away. Imagine this is happening, right now, to you. And now I need your cooperation. I need you to be completely silent for the next seven seconds and remember this place you're in—you are a victim of bullying. Be totally silent." While this story is true, and this did happen to me, I felt weird about adding in these extra little details... the collapsing, falling on my face, wiping away my tears... this moment was traumatic enough as it was; I didn't think my trauma needed more shock value, but this was showbiz now, so I guessed it did.

And just like that, the entire stadium of students and teachers fell SILENT, just as Dick had hoped. And then, something no one in the audience could have expected happened... everything went dark. Every single light in that massive space was turned off, and that's when I opened my mouth to speak once again.

"There's something I haven't told you yet that is my reality. I am blind. [PAUSE] I am COMPLETELY blind!" I remember feeling weird about this because I can still see light and shadow, but I knew that the world thought of blindness as one thing and one thing only: black, dark, nothingness. If they knew I could see something, no matter how little that something might be, then maybe they would think I was lying, faking it, or that everything I had experienced wasn't really all that bad after all. This thought didn't feel so far-fetched because that's how I was treated by my classmates and teachers the very year this took place. I find even now as I'm writing this, I feel a need to justify myself because of decades of having my very existence as a disabled woman invalidated.

Besides, when I wrote and practiced this speech I was in a dimly lit room where I COULDN'T see my hand in front of my face. It was only now, with these incredibly bright stage lights in front of me, that I could see the outline of my hand. But even knowing this, and the fact that in the medical sense, I pretty much am considered fully blind due to having no "functional" vision, I still felt like somehow I was deceiving these people. The doctor no longer asked me to call out the letters I saw, line by line. I could no longer see enough for them to tell me what percentage of my visual field remained or where I fell on the twenty-over-whatever scale. They took pictures of the back of my eye to track the deterioration and that was it. So... was it really a lie? I didn't feel good about it, but in that moment, I'd do anything for a little self-preservation.

After revealing my blindness in a darkened stadium, I wrapped up my speech and invited my guide dog, Gypsy, to the stage to guide me off, which became another unexpected and magical moment for the audience to enjoy. She did exactly as she was told and ran onto the stage, tail wagging, to collect me. She even did a bow, thinking the standing ovation was for her. She was always confident, always a princess, always an attention-seeking, diva-dog extraordinaire, so I was not surprised.

While I was on cloud nine, proud of my performance, I was still surprised to learn that my speech was voted the most impactful at the event. At the end of the six-hour show, students and teachers in attendance filled out a form ranking the performers, and I, little old me, Molly Burke, won the top spot. Huge names like Al Gore, Martin Sheen, and Nelly Furtado had also given speeches and performances... but I was the favorite. For the first time in my entire life, I was popular, and it felt really, really good.

Being popular with the audience meant I was popular with Dick and Sharon. "You should be so pleased with yourself! You were amazing up there, just like we knew you would be!" I'd impressed, I'd made them happy, I'd done my job well. It felt like a test, and I had passed with flying colors. I was ready for phase two.

I was whisked away into another boardroom, this time with the PR team. I was trained on what to say, how to act, and most importantly, how to not embarrass myself or Evolving as One. They had me study celebrity media interviews, quizzing me, "What did Demi do wrong here?" We drilled practice interviews, and they prepared me for every possible situation, from a thirty-second live TV interview to a four-hour conversation with a probing newspaper journalist. Once they felt confident in my ability to perform not just onstage, but in the media, they threw me into every opportunity they could. I was speaking to donors, press, corporations, and at every single pre-party, after-party, and event there was.

I was immediately thrust into a six-week speaking tour where I was expected to do up to ten speeches a week, some just a few minutes long, others an entire hour. I was flying city to city, country to country; from Vancouver to Montreal, then Seattle and Chicago. Canada to America, back to Canada, then back to America again. I was going to after-parties where I sipped on free cocktails, sometimes having a few too many, but it helped me relax and unwind from the chaos. I enjoyed finger foods while signing autographs and taking pictures with strangers who told me they loved me. It was all I'd ever wanted... until it wasn't.

By week five of six, it had been so nonstop that it felt like no amount of sleep would ever be enough. But I knew I could push through. **Just one more week.** At first we had been put up in a dingy motel in downtown San Francisco that reeked of marijuana with walls so thin we could hear the fight that was happening in the adjacent room and the near-constant police sirens from the streets below. After we'd begged to be moved, they actually listened and we arrived in Palo Alto, a wealthy suburb outside of San Fran where we would be staying for the final ten days of my tour. We were in the guest room at a mansion owned by a family who supported a lot of EAO's initiatives, and they were willing to take us in. I was so happy I could cry, not just to get out of that sketchy motel, but to be in a home again that felt warm and inviting.

I'd been bouncing around from shitty hotel to shittier motel. I was exhausted, my throat was sore, and I missed hugging someone who wasn't a random teenager approaching me after I'd done a speech at their middle school. Don't get me wrong, I absolutely adore meeting young people who feel moved or emotionally impacted by my story and giving them a hug. But those hugs are for them ... I'm comforting them in their time of need. Right then, I needed comfort. I needed a mom around, and I needed a day off. I couldn't keep repeating the same forty-five-minute speech over and over and over again like a perfect little robot.

I managed to choke down a few bites of my pumpkin spice bagel before throwing it back up on the floor of a fancy café. I popped another cold and flu tablet in my mouth and called my boss. "Sharon, I need to come home," I told her weakly, then cleared the phlegm from my throat. I felt a stabbing pain whenever I swallowed, I had no appetite, and I was shivering cold, even in the California sun. I just needed to be in my own bed with the love of my mom as she made me her famous homemade Irish chicken stew.

"You can't." Sharon was blunt, using a tone void of emotion.

"Then, can I at least go see a doctor?" I was becoming increasingly concerned that strep throat was to blame for how I was feeling, and if so, I needed antibiotics, like . . . yesterday. She reminded me that I didn't have health insurance through EAO because I hadn't completed my three-month probationary period yet. They also hadn't bothered to purchase me any US travel insurance. Calling around, I found out it would be $800 just to walk in the door of an urgent care as an uninsured traveler, and on my salary—which, at this pace, was starting to feel like just $5 an hour—that was a no go. I can think of a million things EAO probably could've done to help, but evidently none came to their minds. The best thing Sharon was able to do was conjure up one day off. My next two speeches were canceled, and thankfully, my socialite host mom had a doctor friend who agreed to give me an off-the-clock checkup. No strep, but I had a virus of some sort from being so run-down, no doubt caught on one of many flights. I needed to rest, to take a break from a schedule more intense than I realized I had signed up for.

I was no stranger to being sick. In fact, I'd often been very ill as a child. Aside from frequently feeling nauseated, I'd also spend all the fall and winter months going from one sickness to another. If there was a bingo card for infections, viruses, and flus, I'd win every time. After a childhood of antibiotics and over-the-counter meds, days or even weeks of missed school, and countless boxes of tissues and complaints of stomach pain, my parents and I were done with it. With their help, I dedicated myself to getting healthy, and we tried everything we could think of to achieve this, from acupuncture and osteopathy to a low-inflammation, gluten-free, dairy-free diet, herbal medicine, and more. You name it, we probably tried it.

But suddenly, all of these health and wellness practices that had been working to keep illness at bay for the past four years were no longer doing the trick. My mind and body were no match for the rigorous expectations of this job.

I'LL DO ANYTHING

Three months in, I'd passed my probationary period and finally had access to that sweet, sweet corporate health insurance. More importantly, though, I was continuing to crush it at my job and impress everyone around me. So much so that Dick invited me back into that very same boardroom where he had once critiqued me until I reached his level of perfection. But this time, he presented me with the offer of a lifetime. "I want you to write a book," he said. And with a straightforward, no-nonsense tone, he continued on, "Well, let's be honest, you probably won't have time to write a book while you're on the road, so we'll hire you a cowriter."

"What does that mean?" I managed to ask, trying to clarify this literary language that was foreign to me.

"It's basically a ghostwriter, but her name will be on the cover next to yours. She'll conduct a series of interviews with you, spending time getting to know you, your family, your life, and will write the book based on that, with you providing your feedback." Stunned, not having expected something like this would come so soon into my employment, I stammered,

"I... wow! I don't know what to say, this is amazing! Thank you. But do you feel like this is the right time? I feel like I'm still getting used to being on the road so much and adjusting to my new life. I don't know if I can add another thing to my plate, even with a cowriter. It feels like a lot. It's amazing, but a lot right now." I was trying to be as honest as possible while still showing my gratitude to not upset Dick.

"Look," he sighed, "if you don't do this, I'm afraid you won't continue to be as successful here as you could be." **Got it, loud and clear, Dick.**

I wanted to jump for joy, but on the other hand I felt completely overwhelmed. All my wildest dreams were coming true... or so I thought. Looking back, it's hard to know if writing a book really ever was my dream or if it's just something I was told should be. I think we can all agree that writing a book, whether biographical or fictional, is an aspirational idea, but I'll never really know if I would have wanted to do it if I hadn't been told so many times throughout my life, "Wow, you have to write a book someday!" I heard it from teachers, family and friends, and even random strangers who only knew just a tidbit of my story.

"Oh my god, oh my god! You are not going to believe this!" I screamed on the phone to my parents as I raced through the front door of my apartment. I could hardly believe it myself. I was just eighteen years old and getting my first book deal. I only wished I could go back just four years and tell my depressed fourteen-year-old self that one day she'd take all those challenges and channel it into helping others, just the way she'd always wanted to. But just as quickly as the joy came, reality set in.

"I have to advise that you don't sign it." The lawyer my dad hired to review the contract told me that under no circumstances could she in good faith tell me that this was a good deal. And actually, she confirmed, it was a terrible one. Completely "one-sided" is what she said, benefitting no one but Evolving as One. They'd own every right to me, my story, and my likeness till death and ten more years after. They could sell my story and turn it into a movie, a television show, or even a Broadway play. As cool as it sounded to think of **Molly Burke: The Musical!**, giving up all rights to my own life, my own self, didn't seem fair. Despite that, I still wanted to write the book. I didn't feel like I really had a choice. "You won't continue to be as successful here as you could be" were the words that raced through my mind whenever I considered the alternative. Being successful had made me feel like I was worthy, I was valuable, I was enough... I was somebody and I wasn't ready to let that go. I wanted it more than I had ever wanted anything. Ever.

"If you don't let me sign the contract, I'll kill myself, because I'll have nothing to live for anymore and all of my dreams will die with me!" I pleaded with my mom while in an emotional spiral. I paced back and forth, back and forth, leaving footprints in the carpet of my living room. She sat on the couch, stunned by this admission and by the panic that was so evident in my body language and shaky tone. She knew that I had contemplated ending my life in the spring of my eighth-grade year, but thankfully, my dad and she had recognized the warning signs and got me the help that I desperately needed at the time. My parents never stigmatized mental illness, therapy, or treatment to me, and so I had never stigmatized or hidden it myself. I never felt ashamed of my previous suicidal ideation or years of therapy because I was always taught to view it as a normal part of full-body wellness. Just like the common cold or a broken arm. I'm grateful my parents instilled in me such a progressive view of mental health because it's allowed me to always be open with others about where I'm at emotionally. But for the past few years, I'd been in a much better headspace mentally, so hearing me say something like this again came completely out of left field.

I wasn't actively suicidal at the time, but once your mind allows itself to go to the deep, dark thought that ending your life is a valid option, it's easier to let it go there again. Once that door has been opened all the way, it's hard to fully close it for good. People say that suicide is selfish, and while I understand why someone might feel that way, when I was struggling with suicidal thoughts it actually felt like the very opposite. In my mind, Molly was already dead and gone, and what remained was simply a physical body that needed to be cared for. I was a burden on all those around me who still loved me, and there were very few of them. I was a shell of a human, with everything that made me ME already stripped away by vision loss, bullies, and depression. If I were to go, it was far from selfish... it would actually be selfless—I'd be giving them a gift by removing this deadweight from their lives. Once I had decided that ending my life was probably what was best for everyone, I felt more at peace than I had in a very long time. My final parting gift to my family was to make their life easier by leaving it.

I understand that this sounds sick and twisted, and it is. I was sick, and so is everyone else who finds themselves in this cold, lonely place. When having this conversation with my mom, I wasn't trying to use my suicidal past as a manipulative weapon, although I see now that that is exactly what I was doing. But at the time, I genuinely believed that if I didn't get to write this book, I'd disappoint Dick and Sharon, two people who had shown me they believed in me. I'd lose my job and thus I'd no longer have the purpose I lived for in the first place. I didn't want to become a part of that unemployment statistic I'd spent my whole life fearing. **What if this is my only chance?**

And so with the little negotiation that Dick would tolerate, I signed a (slightly) better contract.

THE MOUSE THAT BROKE THE CAMEL'S BACK

By the time the new year rolled around, Gypsy and I were well settled into our life of living alone. While on my lunch break, I sat down on the chocolate-brown Ikea couch that came with the apartment and dug into a freshly made spinach salad. Then I heard it... a noise coming from my stainless-steel kitchen sink.

Is the tap dripping? I thought to myself, standing up to walk over and investigate.

As I got closer, the sound became clearer. Paws. It sounded like tiny little paws were racing around in there.

"I THINK I HAVE A MOUSE!" I shouted to my coworkers as I ran back into our shared office. "Don't be dramatic!" Rebecca calmly reminded me that she lived just below me and if I had a mouse, she would likely also have a mouse, but she didn't. So surely, I didn't either. If only that was how the minds of mice worked.

Ten minutes later we were back in my apartment and realized that she was wrong. Oh so very wrong. The droppings on my kitchen floor and even the countertops were obvious to anyone who could see. Rebecca backtracked and immediately confirmed my fear: "Yup, I'm afraid it's a mouse... and looks like more than just one."

In the coming weeks I'd be awakened in the night by the sound of mice rummaging through my nightstand. I'd stick my hand into my basket of bath bombs, only to feel a mouse race by my fingers. My mom would find six dead mice who had gotten themselves trapped in a bucket in my laundry room, and even Gypsy would find herself face-to-face with a mouse who bravely jumped into her bowl of kibble one morning before she had a chance to take her first bite. After three exterminators, everything reeked of dead mice as their little corpses lay trapped behind my walls. Many were dying, but even more were moving in from the restaurant next door that was mid-renovation. They needed to escape the winter cold, and my cozy home was just the right spot. These were big, bold, city mice who weren't scared of anyone or anything, which is more than I can say for myself.

"I CAN'T DO THIS ANYMORE! YOU NEED TO COME GET ME! I CAN'T STAY HERE!" I shrieked to my parents over the phone, while I stood, shaking in horror, in the middle of my bed where I'd stay, unwilling to put my feet on the floor again until they drove down to escort me to safety.

I didn't have to see the mice to know that they were taking over every inch of my apartment, and I worried that with every step I took, I'd meet another mouse and not even know it. Remember that game we'd play at Halloween parties as children where you'd stick your hand through the hole in a dark box and guess what was inside? Usually, it was cooked spaghetti made to feel like mushy zombie brains or dead worms. This was the adult version of that game, and much less fun. But as fate would have it, I wouldn't have to worry about those mice for much longer...

"You have to move out by the end of the month. We're turning your apartments into an office." Rebecca and I read the email sent from HR while sitting in our shiny silver rental car in the parking lot of Pinkberry. We were on our most recent trip to Northern California, far away from the mice that had invaded my apartment (and then found their way down to hers). "What the hell do they expect us to do?" we wondered aloud. "We're a million miles away from home. We're so busy with all these work trips. How are we going to find the time to prepare and move out?"

"It's like giving someone a birthday gift and then taking it back when you change your mind and decide you want to keep it." We yelled back and forth, angry and frustrated. We had grown tired of their treatment, which felt like less than we deserved and were disillusioned by the "good guy" façade that had once fooled us. It was starting to feel like a disingenuous act, a play they put on to trick the loyal fans into following their every command. In reality, they might just be more shady than authentic, bad actors, as they say.

Some people are willing to do and risk anything to succeed, and it seemed like the execs at EAO were those kinds of people. This whole apartment situation was the straw that broke the camel's back, but there were many more like it. Almost too many to count, like when they strongly encouraged me and Rebecca to drive through a record-breaking snowstorm on my nineteenth birthday to get to a speaking engagement.

What's usually a two-hour drive turned into a dangerous six-hour highway nightmare. Rebecca told me there was no visibility. **Welcome to my life, Rebecca.** "The snow's coming down faster than the wipers can clear it." I could hear the anxiety in her voice over the sound of the news on the radio reporting another crash. Everybody was driving at a snail's pace, not to mention, the road hadn't been plowed, so if your car didn't have all-wheel drive, you were screwed. At this point, we stopped listening to the stressful radio reports, opting for Taylor Swift's **Red** album instead (would recommend in a crisis).

Once we arrived, we discovered that the majority of the audience was unable to attend due to road closures and transit shutdowns. In that moment, we really felt like there was a lack of concern for our safety and well-being. It appeared they cared more about their reputation and profits.

And now that my apartment was going to be more profitable as an office, especially since exterminators finally seemed to get the issue under control, of course EAO wanted the space back. Ugh. And obviously they somehow found the budget to rip up the old, stained carpets, paint the walls a fresh white, and add new can lights—all changes they had insisted were impossible, like when we dared ask if they'd be open to adding better lighting. With the little remaining light perception I have, a few more high hats would've made a big difference in helping me navigate. Oh well. Again, it was their prerogative and as unfair and unkind as it felt, they had every right to make decisions like this. When we asked which staff housing they planned to move us to, they informed us that they didn't have any other suitable units available. Thankfully, they gave me a budget, and with a bit of hunting on the evenings and weekends, followed by their approval, I moved into a five-hundred-square-foot studio apartment above a Tim Hortons, just three blocks from the office.

It was tiny and always too hot, even in the dead of winter (and that's coming from someone who's usually cold). But it was mine and I loved it. I didn't have money for new furniture, so they allowed me to take the furniture from my old apartment with me. After all, they didn't need it anymore now that the accounting department would be working at desks in my old bedroom. Just as I was settling in, another bomb got dropped on me.

"I'm leaving, Molls. I gave it a lot of thought, but once this year is up, I'm going back to work at the school board again."

"WHAT? Are... are you serious? Is there any way you'd consider staying?" While the original plan was that I'd only have Rebecca with me for my first year of work, she had been talking about asking to extend her leave as a vision itinerant, or even quitting entirely so she could continue working with me at EAO. This was the first I was hearing that she had made a final decision, and our time together was going to come to an end. I couldn't even begin to imagine doing all of this without Rebecca by my side. She'd supported me through my final two years of high school, sat with me through a five-hour tattoo session when I got inked for the first time, sweated next to me in countless hot yoga classes, and weathered storm after storm with me over the past year of working at EAO. These sudden changes were becoming too much to bear.

Being my assistant is more than just answering emails and organizing flights, and Rebecca understood that better than almost anyone could. Spending her entire career working with blind people, she knew all the little things, tiny ways to help make my life easier—things that can't just be listed out as tasks in a job description. It's vulnerable allowing someone in to help me with not only work-related things, but life-related things. Inevitably, when you spend so much time on the road together, even sharing a hotel room, the line between work and life gets blurry. (Yes, that's right. EAO made me and my assistant share a hotel room on all of our travels so they could save money.) This type of relationship requires trust, empathy, compassion, and a genuine human connection that can't be forced or manufactured. Those things are hard enough to find organically, and now I had to hope we could hire someone who checked all the boxes and then some. Plus, I was going to miss having someone I could truly call a friend.

This job was hard enough as it was. Could I handle it without her? Would we find the right fit to replace her? I asked myself these questions knowing there was no right person to replace her, but ready or not, it would soon be time to find out, because Rebecca's contract would end in less than two months. What on earth was I going to do?

LOVE BOMBING, GASLIGHTING, AND NEGGING, OH MY!

"Don't hire jessica." We all made it very clear...CRYSTAL CLEAR...so clear that even I could see it. My mom, Rebecca, and I all begged them to hire Joy, the adorable British girl who was as joyful as her name. She already worked in the speaker's department booking events and engagements, and more importantly, we had a great relationship. As soon as she found out that Rebecca was leaving, she applied for the job, only for Sharon to express what is in my opinion a wildly sexist and outdated view with her: "I don't think it would be best for your new marriage if you're traveling and on the road all the time." Despite the fact that Joy assured her that her husband was supportive of her career goals, Sharon was having none of it.

They decided to hire Jessica instead, because why should I get a say in who my assistant would be? It wasn't like I'd have to put all of my trust in this person, regularly share a hotel room, and spend countless hours on the road with them...OH, WAIT! I would. But they didn't seem to care that she had no previous work or education experience that made her well qualified for this specific role, and they sure didn't seem to care that we didn't get along well. We had nothing in common, from basic things like our taste in music or food, to deeper things like how we were raised, to big things like the fact that I had a guide dog and Jessica DIDN'T LIKE DOGS! She liked science, I liked fashion. She was introverted, I was extroverted. We were oil and water. It was as if all they wanted in an employee was a brainwashed superfan of the organization and, therefore, someone who would be willing to do anything for the job. Luckily for them, her actions gave the impression that she was one. I heard a rumor that she had already applied to more than twenty different positions at EAO and had driven halfway across the country for the in-person interview. She was willing to do anything it took, put aside personal boundaries, have zero work-life balance, and drop everything to be one of their "change makers," all in the name of saving the world.

I wondered how much positive change was EAO making if they were willing to hurt people like me to achieve it?

While I maybe once held on to this idealistic view of the charitable work we were doing at Evolving as One, I had become indifferent to it after a year of feeling mistreated. I was overworked to the point that I now too was passing weary glances to my equally exhausted coworkers, and with a dull, lifeless expression, I'd mutter the running office joke I'd overheard time and time again, "Devolving as One!"

I knew that to be freed, it would really only take one simple thing: quitting. But as simple as it sounds—and in practice, it would be—it felt harder for me than it should. If I quit, what would my life be like? I was nineteen, living on my own in the city, traveling the world with an assistant, even if it was one that I didn't like all that much. I was in magazines, performing at stadiums, and hanging out with A-listers in greenrooms. On some of the tours, I'd get catered lunches, makeup touch-ups, and invites to open-bar parties. **It doesn't get better than this, right?** But while those were the highlights, the lowlights were low. Dirty motels in sketchy neighborhoods,[6] a daily food allowance that barely afforded the most basic breakfast, lunch, and dinner, and long drives to rural towns performing to an audience of fifty alongside an Elvis impersonator. I was having my personal boundaries constantly crossed and EAO's "core values" thrown in my face anytime I tried to speak up. "Get the job done, period" was their de facto motto.

I was often expected to travel on weekends, making it impossible to complete typical weekend tasks like laundry or grocery shopping. One time I asked to take a lieu day and, incredulous at the idea, they told me, "Weekend travel days

---

6. Or that one time I stayed in a bed-and-breakfast that used to be the town morgue, so I lovingly refer to it as "The Dead and Breakfast"—although there was no breakfast because all their food was rotten. I guess all things go there to die! I'm so thankful we made it out alive.

don't count." Their average turnover rate was apparently just eight short months, and I'm not surprised because expectations like the ones I was under were not sustainable. Surely most people would crack under that pressure and leave. The bad days were more common than the good, but were the good ones good enough to stay for?

More than anything, though, I was acutely aware that regardless of the bad, I was still one of the lucky ones. I might not have been getting paid much, but I was certainly getting paid more than the government money I could be living on like so many of my disabled friends. So, no matter what, I'd suck it up and wouldn't complain. Besides, anytime someone had the gall to complain about the working conditions, someone in HR or management was quick to remind us that, statistically speaking, it was "harder to get a job at EAO than it is to get into Harvard." I'll never know how true that was, but they loved to say it.

Without Rebecca around, it started feeling like nobody important at work cared about me, and that feeling of isolation really hurt. I used to think Sharon cared, but if she did, I don't think she would have said things like, "You're not that special; don't go getting a big head and become a prima donna!" when I was doing anything but. It was as if the management and executives wanted to keep me down, humble me, make me feel insecure like my former bullies did, so I'd continue to accept what little I was being given. The initial love bombing turned to gaslighting, negging, and the dangling promise of better days. And Jessica was about to prove to me that better days weren't to come with her as my assistant, like on our first trip together, which would be one month in India.

"India" had been my nickname with some people around the office, and I often thought about the fact that if I had the choice, I'd probably change my name and officially be India. Molly, meaning "sea of bitterness," never felt quite right. I think many young people go through this whole "I hate my name" thing, and I have grown into a proud Molly at this point, but my name was so publicly tied to my identity that it was practically synonymous with my "brand," if you could call it that, so I couldn't change it now. Alas, I'd just live with India as my (now-long-lost) nickname. It was coined by a coworker who saw how much I loved and appreciated her Indian culture.

Growing up, I had a mentor named Avina who was like my Indian older sister. She went to a local high school that required a certain number of volunteer hours each year in order to graduate. She somehow got connected with my family and ended up volunteering to help me with my homework after school once a week. She'd force me to read my braille books, which I hated, and we'd practice touch-typing on the computer. But she would also try to break up the boring things I didn't want to do with fun things I did. We'd go to the movies and get ice cream, and then she started to introduce me to the wonderful world of curry, and taught me about Hinduism while doing henna on my arms, and couldn't have been more excited when I began to practice yoga.

I loved Avina, and I loved everything she would tell me about India, and because of that, it was always at the top of my travel bucket list. When EAO asked me if I'd like to spend a month there as a leadership facilitator on one of their youth trips, I jumped at the chance. They'd sell the trip as "a month with Molly," and eager parents would line up to pay thousands of dollars for their teen to have the opportunity to spend one-on-one time with me abroad. No pressure!

Jessica coughed and cleared her throat as we boarded the Air India flight out of the Pearson International Airport in Toronto. "Still sick?" I asked as she blew her nose. I guess that was my answer. For weeks I had been telling my parents and Mark, my onetime YMCA work friend–turned–recent boyfriend, that I didn't want to go to India anymore. "I don't know what it is . . . I just have a bad feeling about it. I'm exhausted, I'm burnt out, and I don't know if I can be everything these kids want me to be." The inner pressure to be for my audience what I had once needed someone to be for me felt immense.

Could the real-life me live up to the version of me they had in their head? Was I good enough or would twenty-four-seven me be a disappointment in comparison to the five-minute or one-hour me they knew from the stage? When you have an audience, big or small, they only see certain aspects of who you are, the parts you choose to share. But when you spend a month with someone, day in and day out, you see all of them. You see the good, even the great. But you also see the very real, human parts that aren't to be placed on a pedestal or admired... the parts of you that get frustrated, feel tired, or just want some alone time. Would they, or could they, love that Molly too? I didn't feel confident enough to find out. I knew deep down that I'd have to try to be "on" the entire time.

They thought it was just nerves, or that perhaps I didn't want to leave now that I was falling madly in love with Mark, or maybe even that I was sad because I had to leave Gypsy behind. They encouraged me to go and assured me, "We'll take good care of Gypsy, Mark will be here when you get home, and remember, you've ALWAYS wanted this." Knowing I couldn't afford to go to India if it wasn't for this work trip, I packed up my hiking backpack with sweatpants, sneakers, and Goldfish crackers, and took my seat on the flight next to a sniffling and snotty Jessica.

After three flights, listening to too many sneezes to count, and a bit of airplane constipation, we finally arrived. The energy as we exited the airport in Udaipur felt ELECTRIC. Any remaining exhaustion from the nearly twenty-four hours of travel melted away with the buzz of the city streets around me. **Jet lag who? I'm ready—let's go explore!** But oh wait, I can't.

I was unable to go anywhere without Jessica's help, and Jessica was unable to lift her head off the hotel pillow. The jet lag (or flu) had gotten to her. I sat on the edge of my bed, twiddling my thumbs, waiting for her to wake up so we could hit the streets and see everything the famous "City of Lakes" had to offer.

Once she was ready, I was beyond ready to make the absolute most of the two full days we had before the twenty teens would arrive with our third facilitator, Chelsea. We took tuk tuks into town and popped in and out of local shops, admiring the beautiful saris and ornate gold jewelry. We took in all the sounds and smells around us as we sipped on masala. We even visited the home of one of our tuktuk drivers—admittedly, going to a stranger's home in a foreign country wasn't the safest choice for two young female travelers to make, but thankfully he was a gentleman!

Things, however, were about to take a turn for the worse. After picking up Chelsea and the bright-eyed and bushy-tailed trip participants, we drove two hours into the rural, middle-of-nowhere Rajasthan, where we'd spend the remainder of our stay. The goal was to help build a school that was being funded by EAO. We'd be working on laying the foundation of the building before the next group arrived to take it from there. That night, what I thought was jet lag finally seemed to hit. **That's odd . . . I've been here for a few days; why am I just now feeling it?** I thought to myself, shivering cold in the humid August evening air.

I immediately knew something was wrong when I woke up in the morning, dripping sweat despite still being freezing cold. I felt a sharp, stabbing pain in my throat, and as I opened my mouth to tell Jessica and Chelsea, still lying in their beds on either side of mine, no sound came out. I'd been sick plenty of times, but never in my whole entire life had I literally been left speechless. Apparently, Jessica hadn't been over her contagious phase after all.

After days of being unable to eat and barely able to squeak out a sound, wincing in pain every time I swallowed, I was put in a car alone with a local driver who didn't speak English. The other facilitators decided it would be better for both Jessica and Chelsea to stay rather than for one to accompany me. Consistently, I felt the people at EAO demonstrated they didn't understand the gravity of my blindness. How could they not realize the vulnerability of being in a foreign country with a stranger who you can't communicate with, unable to see your surroundings, with no phone (the local flip phones for the other facilitators had no screen reader), and nothing but a cane to keep me safe—the mobility aid I wasn't used to using. I wanted to remind them that I was just a year older than some of the trip participants who were definitely not allowed anywhere without a guardian.

The driver brought me two hours back to Udaipur to the closest emergency room where I met a local EAO staff member. I could finally let my guard down again, thinking, **She's got it from here.** Seeing the state of me, the doctors rushed me past the waiting patients to examine me. I was given four different prescriptions. Antibiotics, anti-inflammatories, pain meds, and probiotics. Prescriptions filled, I could begin the road to recovery. Or so I thought...

I'd go the next three weeks bouncing from one infection to another, going to different specialists, and trying out a whole host of meds, all while trying to recover in a permanently damp, mold-filled hotel room with zero hot water. Hardly able to eat because the spice burned my throat and we were too far from the city to access things like cold yogurt to soothe the pain, I was living on bananas, coconut water, and my ever-diminishing Goldfish. I threw up on my favorite, brand-new, mint-green sweatpants from Pink. Not enough food plus too much medication is not a good combo. I was struggling, I was suffering, and I wanted to go home. I was rapidly losing weight, managing to have dropped ten pounds in just a few short weeks. Jessica and Chelsea had to care for the teens, so I was left alone in the hotel for eight to ten hours a day. Built on a mountainside, the hotel grounds were a maze. There were winding, uneven stone paths that were decorated by hundreds of stairs. With few English-speaking staff and no braille signage to help navigate, when they left for the day, I was completely stuck in my room with nothing but what I had. I literally didn't even have a way to call for help if I needed it. And when they arrived home in the evenings, they would burst through the door, turning on all the lights and talking at full volume, ignoring the fact that I was in bed trying to sleep off my illness. I felt invisible.

I weakly asked Jessica to help me use her phone to call home. Unable to use work phones for personal calls, the only person I was able to talk to was Sharon. "I'm too sick to do anything. I can barely even leave my hotel room. I'm hardly hanging out with the kids, they're already not getting the trip they were promised, so nothing will change if I leave!" I started to cry, feeling so lonely and hopeless, "I'm not going to recover here. Every time I think that I'm starting to feel better, I get sick again. My body is run-down. I need to be at home." She informed me that there was no way they could do that, besides, "You'd regret it if you left. Is there anything we can send from home that would help?"

The bunny I had slept with every night since I was born, my favorite peppermint tea, throat lozenges, some protein bars so I wouldn't continue to waste away to nothing...I offered up a whole list. They never sent anything.

FALL FROM GRACE

Upon our return from India, Jessica and I embarked on our first and only speaking tour together, and it was a disaster. Arriving at the airport, Jessica acted flustered and admitted that she forgot her passport, along with an important cord for the computer that would allow my visual presentation to be shown on-screen during my speech, something I did during every event. Thankfully, our first stop on the trip was within Canada so she was still able to board our flight using her driver's license. Another staff member went into her apartment to collect her passport and mail it to the EAO office in Vancouver. It didn't come on time for us to make our flight to Seattle, which forced us to take a 5-hour bus ride (with multiple stops and a transfer) overnight to make it to my next commitment on time.

Once there, I woke up at 4 A.M. to the sound of our hotel door quietly closing, leading me to believe she had just arrived back from the staff after-party. My suspicion deepened when I smelled whiskey on her breath an hour later when we got up to leave for my early-morning television appearance.

On the third stop of the tour, I found myself sick in bed once again, pushed to the limit of what my body could handle (vertigo this time), and I hoped to see some compassion from her. But instead I was left feeling abandoned, her cell phone seemingly dead or left unchecked for what felt like hours on end, leaving me without access to food.

And on one fall night in Minnesota, she vocalized so much hesitation to use the corporate credit card to get us a taxi back to the hotel that we ended up walking home. She said she feared retribution from EAO for exceeding our daily budget, and as much I understood that, I didn't feel safe walking back. After pleading with her to no avail, I lost the argument. She was older, she was sighted, she held the card, and she was supposed to keep me safe. It felt like my only option was to agree to walk the forty-five minutes in the dark, nothing on my feet but tights that were slowly ripping as the asphalt rubbed against them with every step. I had been standing in my black patent Jessica Simpson pumps for far too long at the corporate cocktail party, so shoeless, I walked.

It took more convincing than it should have, but once I finally put my foot down and presented Sharon and HR with a well-documented list of Jessica's mistakes, they moved her to another department, and with no other options to find a quick replacement, Sharon finally agreed to let Joy step in to fill Jessica's very small shoes. Joy was off to a great start. She was warm, friendly, and, most importantly, good at her job. We shared the same taste in television shows, had similar hobbies, and the same dry, sarcastic sense of humor. All was well, until it wasn't.

It was just two weeks after my twentieth birthday when tragedy struck. As per usual those days, I was overworked, drained, and running on empty. Having no control over my schedule, unable to say yes or no to the events they booked for me, this felt like a roller coaster that I couldn't get off. I was motion sick, and I was starting to debate whether the thrills were worth all the discomfort. When you have a life like mine, you learn that things are mostly bad and hard and painful; that's just what it is. You try to hold on to all the good things that make it tolerable because it's the only way to survive. When you're climbing the hill, you're filled with the anticipation, wondering if the drop will be fun, or will it be too much? For me, it's almost always too much, but I kept believing maybe the next time would be different. And maybe it would be ... or maybe I'd crash.

I was doing my sound check, prepping for yet another presentation, just like I had numerous times before. Walking onto the stage to count out how many steps I'd have to work with, I decided to leave Gypsy behind because I like to have both hands free to feel my way around. Joy was already onstage, counting the steps aloud and describing everything as she went so I'd know what to expect. My mind was foggy, and I could only half listen as I walked up behind her.

One step, two steps, three steps. BAM! With her back turned to me, Joy didn't see me approaching the edge of the stage. Full speed ahead, I walked straight off the five-foot drop, landing on the concrete floor below. One of my finest blind girl moments.

I was in shock, unsure of what had happened at first. I heard a gasp, then Joy and the event manager came running. Embarrassed, I insisted, "I'm all right, seriously. Don't worry about it!" even offering up a little laugh for good measure. **That's right, Molly, sell it!** I thought to myself. **Be professional and never let anyone see you when you're down.**

I made a few self-deprecating jokes, the same way I always did. I thought, **If I own my blindness and make fun of myself, then no one else can make fun of me for it because I already have.** This is something I've done for as long as I can remember. Humor is a common coping mechanism I've seen used in my own household. Call it nature or call it nurture, but it's worked for me time and time again. That day was no different.

Ten minutes later, the audience filed in, and I gave two back-to-back, hour-long speeches. **No one in the audience ever has to know.**

"Mom, you'll never guess what I did!" I said, calling my mom on the car ride home. At this point, I was genuinely starting to think it was funny. My hip was bruised and my neck a bit stiff, but all in all, it could have been much worse. "I mean, it was bound to happen eventually, right?!" Not thinking much of it, I bantered back and forth on the phone with Mark about it after hanging up with my mom, who insisted that my dad stop by my apartment on his way home from work to check on me. "I'm fine, seriously, it's not a big deal!" My coaxing didn't sway her. She knew from the life-changing accident that I had when I was nine years old that this likely was, in fact, a big deal.

It was the winter of 2004. I could feel the snow coming down in sheets, blanketing the earth beneath me. The loud call of the bell was ringing in my ears, signaling the end of recess. Racing from the back of the playground to get inside for class, I felt the snow crunch with every step. The entire world looked bright white, lacking any kind of depth or detail. Disoriented and running in the wrong direction, I slipped and smacked my face on something jagged. Amidst the cold whipping winds, a sticky warmth washed over my face as I reached out and felt the edge of a metal fence. In shock, I suddenly felt a hand grab my arm. "Molls, you're bleeding!" It was the voice of my half-friend, half-bully Christina. Not caring that I was getting blood all over her cream snowpants (head wounds truly bleed like no others), she led me down the hall while I tracked gruesome red trails behind us. After multiple failed attempts from the office staff to stop the bleeding, they called my mom. A few stitches to the nose later, and it was official: I had to start using a cane.

That accident shook me to my core, and so would this one; I just didn't know it yet. Funny how sometimes our parents seem to know us better than we know ourselves. After my dad checked in, I started thinking back to the insomnia I'd developed following my previous accident, where I would spend night after night pacing my room, unable to sleep. I wasn't going to let that happen this time. Popping a sleeping pill to ensure a good night's rest after a hectic day, I fell into a deep sleep, only half-aware of the shooting pain running up the side of my neck as I tossed and turned.

My mom used the spare key to let herself into my apartment before I even woke up. Sitting on the couch just five feet from my bed, she noticed the moment my eyes began to flutter open. "How are you feeling?" I heard the concern in her voice. I sat up, the pain hitting me as I realized I couldn't seem to fully turn my neck to look over my left shoulder. **This is definitely worse than I thought.** Off to the ER we went.

Every time my mom would brake at a red light, I'd feel a stabbing pain. I braced myself, just hoping it would hurt a little less. The doctors would tell me that the force of the fall and the angle at which I'd landed had caused me to tear the small ligaments and tissues on the side of my neck. I'd need to wear a foam neck wrap and get physiotherapy. Apparently, the full extent of the pain from muscular damage doesn't present itself for up to forty-eight hours after the injury occurs ... who knew!

Well, now I did. But I also knew that I had to return to work. After I'd rested for a few days, it was time for my first speech back. I was speaking at a local high school during first period, opening with a joke about my new foam fashion accessory. I was halfway through when all of a sudden something strange started to happen... I felt disconnected from my thoughts. I was still saying words, but my mind went blank. All at once, I was frozen, filled with the irrational fear that if I took just a single step, even backward, I'd begin to fall.

Then, with every presentation after, it got worse. My heart would pound before I walked onstage, as if for the first time in my life I experienced what must have been... stage fright? This was something I'd heard of, but never experienced. For me, being onstage came as naturally as breathing itself. So, why was I racing to the bathroom with diarrhea, sweating, dry mouth? I must have been sick.

Weeks went by, and I was hardly able to eat, my stomach in constant knots. I saw doctors, both Western and Eastern, but no one seemed to know the cause of my illness. All packed up and ready to go, sick or not, I had an early-morning flight to catch. I was off to the UK for two weeks where I'd be speaking alongside Malala Yousafzai, Richard Branson, Ellie Goulding, and Evanna Lynch at Wembley Arena for the first-ever major UK event. And I was NOT willing to miss it.

Sure, Prince Harry would be there, and that was cool and all, but I was most excited to see Mark. My boyfriend had been studying abroad in Wales for three months and had three more to go. This would be our one and only chance to see each other during his six months away, and I needed him now more than ever.

My mom had prepared him so he wouldn't be shocked by my frail frame, with my extra-small leggings fitting baggy around the waist. Together, they made a list of what he needed to have ready when I landed: nuts, protein bars, and even a mini blender to make smoothies, one of the few things I could manage to get down.

Desperate for answers, my mom began to Google my symptoms. Shockingly, the first result wasn't cancer, as it usually seems to be when searching ANYTHING medical. As I sat in bed in my darkened room the night before my flight, she read a list from her phone to me. I got animated. "Yes, that's it! That's me! What is it?"

"Post-traumatic stress disorder."

RED FLAGS WAVING

It wasn't my best performance, I'll admit, but I wasn't expecting it to be. I was just trying to get through it with a smile on my face. It's just like EAO always reiterated, "Don't ask yourself if you can. Ask yourself how you will."

Everyone at work was aware of my fragile state, demonstrated by my inability to get through a staff dinner on our first night in London without running to the bathroom to have what I now know was a panic attack. Day by day, it was getting worse, not better. "Would it be all right if someone else took over for me at the after-party?" Willing to do my most important engagements, I was only asking to be removed from speaking at the events that any of their other speakers were equally capable of doing. After I sent the email, my phone rang. It was Joy, busy at the venue, preparing for the big day.

"Hey, what's up?" I tried to sound casual while my heart pounded in my chest. I loved and trusted Joy; she was always on my side and made me feel supported. I really felt like she had my best interests at heart like Rebecca had. But I still got nervous at the thought of anything work-related, and anything Joy would be calling about was undoubtably work-related.

"Hi, Molly!" The voice in my ear was familiar but it wasn't Joy... **What? Why on earth is one of Dick's executives calling me on my assistant's phone? Is this some sort of prank call?** Red flags waving, I tried to remain cool. "Oh, hey, good to hear from you! Is everything all right?" That's when I was informed that if I chose not to speak at any engagement they had planned for me, I'd have to pay for the hotel room myself.

All right, I see how it is. You don't care about me, my well-being, my mental or physical health. You don't care about me unless I'm making you money, but the moment I have a workplace accident and can't perform at my peak, I'm useless and no longer matter. In that moment, everything was so clear to me. All of the excuses that I had been making to justify how they treated me vanished. They were all lies I had been telling myself so that I could hold on to the dream that Dick had sold me that spring evening at Starbucks two years earlier.

I paid for a new hotel room for my final night and notified the team that my pre-booked one-week vacation was officially beginning early and they shouldn't expect to receive replies to any emails. I was done. They had finally pushed me to my breaking point.

That night, I sat in bed with Mark and ate an entire pizza.

My cognitive behavioral therapist would be the one to officially give me the formal diagnosis. "Complex PTSD," he'd say, in a matter-of-fact kind of way. Almost as if I should have known all along, he explained to me that, while this most recent accident had triggered my current episode, he believed this CPTSD had been haunting me for a very long time. Suddenly, it felt like so many dots in my life were being connected. I hadn't needed a two-night sleep study when I was nine; I'd needed therapy. I didn't need anti-nausea meds; I needed ones for anxiety.

He told me then and there, "You can choose to keep working and injure your brain long-term, or you can choose to step away for a bit and work on healing it." Nodding, I stuck my hand out as he passed over the doctor's note I'd require for my six-week medical leave.

Forced to bring the note to Sharon and Dick, I was filled with dread: **Would they be mad at me? How many people was I going to disappoint or let down?** But even more than that worry, I was overcome with a sense of relief. I was getting exactly what, deep down, I knew I needed and wanted but didn't have the courage to decide for myself.

My parents would help me pack up my apartment and drive everything back to my childhood home in the suburbs. I'd continue with cognitive behavioral therapy as well as talk therapy. I'd learn about coping techniques like box breathing and the physical mechanics of what was really happening to my mind and body during my all-too-frequent anxiety attacks.

My therapist had been seeing me on and off since I was just thirteen, and she knew me inside and out. "You'll never be happy there, Molly." Her voice was honest, kind... "You lack so much control in your life already, not being able to see the world around you... It's important that you have control in other aspects of your life, like work. Unless and until they're willing to give that to you, you won't be happy." I sighed, knowing she was right. My time was up.

Sitting across from one of EAO's top execs, the head of HR, and Sharon, I looked over at them with a blank expression and lifeless eyes. "I can only give what I have, and I have given you everything. It's time for me to give to myself again for a while." They feigned care and compassion for what felt like the first time, but I'm fairly certain it wasn't real and that they were just as happy I'd be gone as I was. Finally, I felt free. Free from the pressure, the judgment, the unrealistic expectations, and their sly remarks.

In the following weeks we'd exchange some wrap-up emails and phone calls, getting everything squared away. My upcoming book tour would be postponed, and later canceled—something I'd thought would crush me but actually felt more like a weight had been lifted. My book, **Through My Eyes: Blind and Bullied but Not Broken**, would never see the light of day, and thank god for that. While writing a book initially felt like a dream come true, the reality is that I barely played a part in its creation, and by the time it was complete I hated nearly everything about it. Much like most of the work I did with EAO, it felt rushed, forced, and less authentic than I wanted it to be. It didn't exactly feel like it, but maybe it would all work out for the best if I just kept my head above water.

The stress of it all wasn't just impacting me, it seemed to be affecting Gypsy as well. While I was dealing with my neck injury and CPTSD on my medical leave and navigating quitting my job and moving back home, Gypsy was fighting a battle of her own. At first I noticed she was a little gassy—no big deal, hot girls have stomach problems, right? But in the coming weeks, her symptoms rapidly progressed. It was clearly more than sympathy sickness; she wasn't finishing the food in her bowl, the vomiting became more frequent, and so did the vet visits.

When the symptoms were mild, the vet suspected she had just eaten something nasty in the city streets as the winter snow began to melt and uncover all the secrets that lay beneath. But the special gastrointestinal food and antacids weren't helping. We did blood work, checked her urine, and did a stool sample. "It's all clean... Everything looks normal," the vet said. I should have felt relief hearing this news, but deep down inside I knew something was seriously wrong. As her health continued to decline, I pushed for answers: "What more can we do?" To which the vet suggested it was time for an X-ray.

The X-ray would reveal a large blockage in her intestine. "Is it possible that she ate a toy, or a sock?" my vet asked. "No, she doesn't do stuff like that... She's a highly trained guide dog... She'd never do that." While guide dogs do have their flaws, I knew she wouldn't pick up such a bad habit at nine and a half years old. "Well, you never know," she responded, before explaining, "it could be something like a doggy Crohn's disease, or..." She paused, and I could tell she didn't want to continue. I held my breath as she delivered the blow: "It could be cancer."

While cancer was unlikely, the only way to know for sure was to perform an exploratory surgery. I felt I understood the torture that my parents went through watching me go undiagnosed and having exploratory tests and surgeries of my own. Gypsy wasn't my child, but it felt like she was. Even more than that, she felt like a piece of me... an extension of my own being. She saw what I could not. And for seven years she'd walked on my left side, keeping me safe, giving me confidence, and making me feel less alone in the darkness of what felt like so much isolation. She'd been with me for the vision loss, the depression, and the bullying. She'd been my constant in an ever-changing reality. Switching schools, graduating, and attending prom. My first love, followed by my first heartbreak—she was there for it all. Moving out, traveling the world—we hit these milestones together. But now I was forced to face the reality I had long refused to believe: she wouldn't be there by my side forever.

The surgery revealed that it was worse than the worst-case scenario. It was cancer, a five-inch tumor in her bowel, and it had already spread throughout her body. "We can remove seven inches of her bowel and stitch her back up, but she'd likely only have a few weeks to live. Or we can just leave her sleeping." When I asked about the quality of those few weeks, I was told that she'd continue to go downhill. I made probably the hardest decision I ever have. "Can I come see her to say goodbye?" As much as I wanted to hold on, I knew that keeping her alive would be for me, while letting her go and be free from the misery that her life had become would be the last gift I could give her.

My parents and I rushed to see her. The fifteen-minute drive felt never-ending. Despondent, I sat in shock in the back seat. I heard my parents trying to talk to me, but none of their words made sense. All I could focus on was the sound of her favorite lizard toy as I held it, remembering the last time I heard her squeak it. I never thought when I dropped her off that I wouldn't see her awake again. I wished I'd thanked her. She deserved a better goodbye.

Standing in the sterile operating room, I reached for Gypsy's soft ear, still warm, to rub against my cheek one final time. My family and the vet watched from the hallway as I whispered to her, "I love you..." I didn't know if she heard the pain in my voice or knew how much I would miss her. I sobbed, holding her paw in my hand as she lay on a cold metal table, blanket wrapped around her. I felt her chest rise and fall as the tube extending from her mouth breathed for her.

I soaked up every last moment with her. I was so grateful for everything she'd done for me, and I was heartbroken that I never got to tell her, "I am who I am because of you." They pulled me from the room.

Those words were true. She gave me joy when it was hard to feel, strength in the face of so many storms, and the freedom to live the life I wanted despite my vision loss. Most people will never understand how one dog could do that for someone, but that's just the tip of the iceberg (or should I say, tip of the tail) of what she did for me.

Losing her felt like losing a piece of myself all over again. My world was crumbling down around me, and I didn't know how to keep going. Everything that I had worked so hard to rebuild after vision loss—my health, my happiness, my independence... It was all gone. I had the strength to overcome it once, but I didn't feel like I had it in me to do it a second time. No job, no apartment in the city, and most devastating, no Gypsy. The one who was with me, by my side through it all, had left me, and I felt more alone than ever.

Wrapped up in the hand-knitted blanket my aunt made for me, I'd curl in a ball and cry on the bathroom floor for hours. Sometimes my thoughts would race, flashing through my mind again and again. Other times, it seemed like I couldn't follow a single thought through to completion. My dad found me sitting at the top of the stairs in my teddy bear pajamas, hands gripping each side of my head. "My brain is broken, my brain is broken!" I'd repeat, rocking back and forth with tears streaming down my cheeks.

My body felt like a living torture chamber. I wanted to escape and be anywhere but here. Anywhere but inside this body that houses this brain that won't let me sleep and won't let me eat. I felt trapped, not only in my body but in my life. Was this really who I was supposed to be? How had it gotten this bad again? How had I gotten here?

I'd visit a psychiatrist, who'd give me my first SSRI prescription to combat the anxiety that had overtaken my mind, body, and life. He'd tell me that what I was experiencing were "OCD tendencies" accompanying my CPTSD and generalized anxiety disorder. The four panic attacks a day would soon turn to three, then two, then none. With my mind relaxing, my body could relax too, and I enjoyed drinking all the chocolate milkshakes and eating all the mac and cheese I could to help put back on the weight that had been falling off me for months. The fog in my brain was lifting, and the therapy was working... I was starting to uncover the answers to so many questions.

As I grew to understand myself better, I also grew to forgive myself for letting it get to this point. I now knew what a perfect target I was for what some would call this "cult" where I had been working for nearly two years. After a lifetime of bullying, what felt like workplace abuse was nothing new to me. Their ill treatment of me was familiar, and I handled it the same way I always had: stay quiet, avoid confrontation, and people-please my way out of it. I was used to having my personal life and trauma on public display for the gain of others; in a way, Ending Blindness had been doing something similar to me since I was five years old and too young to truly consent. My parents, brainwashed by an ableist world, were convinced that the only way to be good parents to their blind daughter was to find her a cure. I don't blame them; I blame cure culture and the world that dangled it as hope.

As I craved acceptance, the feeling of fitting in and being liked... it felt good. I was impressionable and willing to do anything, just trusting it was the right thing, no matter how wrong it felt. I was lucky. I should be grateful. So many other talented and deserving disabled people weren't getting opportunities like this, so how could I give it up? When you've never known better, you don't expect better. You accept what you're given, what you think you deserve.

Some say let the past be the past, but the truth is, it's never that easy. In many ways, our past does define us. It forms who we are and influences the choices we make, the opinions we hold, the triggers we have. I've spent years unlearning and relearning, unpacking decades of buried memories to understand exactly how I got here.

FADE TO BLACK

In the fall of 2008, I was in my second year at a fancy private school, surrounded by girls who, on the weekends, wore Juicy Couture sweats while carrying their Louis Vuitton purses and glossing their lips with MAC Cosmetics, desperately clutching their signature Tiffany heart necklaces, knowing that they were, in fact, THAT girl. Two years prior, I had read the **Clique** series, or rather, my mom had read it aloud to me, since it hadn't yet existed as an audiobook. These girls I now found myself surrounded by were just like Massie and Alicia—wealthy, pretty, worldly, and popular—and I was their Claire—less cool and sophisticated in every way possible. It felt like I was living the real-life **Gossip Girl**, sitting in class next to the Blair Waldorfs and Serena van der Woodsens of the world, and I wasn't even a Jenny Humphrey. If this was real-world **Mean Girls**, I was Cady Heron . . . just an outsider trying to fit in with a group of girls who felt so foreign to everything I was used to (okay, I'll stop with all of my early 2000s pop culture references, but . . . if you get it, you get it!).

I wasn't like them—my family couldn't afford the same things. Don't get me wrong, I was not hard done by. I grew up upper-middle-class with a hardworking dad and a creative, entrepreneurial mom. They did anything and everything they could to give my brother and me a comfortable life, and they had succeeded. We lived in a beautiful redbrick home that they renovated after my diagnosis to make sure that we'd have big windows to let in natural light, and can lights with dimmer switches throughout so I could always make it bright enough to see or dark enough when my eyes hurt. They repainted my room in more vivid and high-contrast colors when my vision inevitably changed and the light green began to look white, or later, when I could no longer see the difference between the pink and orange hues. We had a pool in the backyard and a basketball net in the driveway. We had nice things, but not as nice as these girls'. We went on vacation every four or five years, but they had vacation homes. My mom dropped me off each morning in a used Jeep packed with her gardening gear, while their moms drove the latest BMWs and Mercedes ... you get it. When I could see enough to fake my way, I was fine, but the moment the world began to fade away even more, things got much harder.

My older brother was already a star pupil, having entered the school two years earlier when he was in seventh grade. Too smart and talented to sit still in his previous public school classes, he needed an environment that would challenge him to reach his full potential, and that's exactly what this school provided. He was popular, got straight A's, took multiple languages like French and Mandarin, played sports, and was in the school musical. He was a well-rounded, high-achieving kid, which was exactly what the school expected in a student. Once they found out that his little sister was blind, they immediately asked my parents if I'd like to attend in the fall. I didn't even have to sit the two-day academic assessment or go through the interview process required of the other hopefuls. They took a look at my previous report cards and school records, and just like that, I was in.

The school grounds were large, old, and beautiful, with a rich history. Surrounded by a forest, the property backed onto a wide, sweeping river that cut through the landscape like a four-lane highway. The architecture had a British charm. It felt like going to school at Hogwarts but with a lot less magic.

Set up like a college campus, it had a grand dining hall, a swimming pool next to both the tennis and squash courts, a drama theatre that Shakespeare himself would've been proud of, and a boathouse for our renowned sailing team. There were multiple dormitory buildings, some for boys and some for girls, where all seniors and the international students lived. It was a combination of middle and high school, and all students HAD to live on campus during their final year. They said it was to prepare us for when we'd go away to university, but I suspect it was just another way to make more money and charge a higher tuition.

I don't know what they were using that extra money for though, because it certainly didn't seem to be for accessibility. The campus lacked any kind of wheelchair-friendly ramps, elevators, or doors. I expected a private school might be elitist, but I'm sure even they understood that they couldn't risk being called out publicly for being discriminatory, so rather than make expensive and time-consuming structural adjustments, they must have thought that admitting one blind girl could be a quick and easy fix to look more inclusive. Said blind girl was, in fact, not me—I came later. Funny enough, it was that very same little girl who my mom had seen on the cover of our local newspaper all those years earlier on the day of my diagnosis.

Maeve was now a confident redhead with an adorable guide dog, Marble. She and her younger brother, Finn, were both blind from birth. They were quiet, but they were brilliant, both of them. But being blind from birth is very different than my reality. When they'd learned to read, they'd done it with braille. When they'd learned to use a computer, it was with a screen reader. They never saw colors, or faces, or ... anything. Blindness was the only life they'd ever known. Me, on the other hand ... I was living in the middle. Not quite sighted, not quite blind. My vision had been changing throughout my childhood: I was fully blind at night or in dim lighting but able to see pretty well during the day or in well-lit environments. I could read large print, then larger, and then even larger. I could use ZoomText, a program that allows you to enlarge anything on the computer, and different features to see and navigate the screen more easily. I could see colors, though they were beginning to fade and blend more and more with time. Black looked gray, and all pastel colors melted into white. My world was changing, and I was continually having to adapt.

I'm not here to argue whether being born blind or going blind is harder. They both have their own unique benefits and hardships, and frankly, I'm not really interested in participating in the Oppression Olympics. I simply share this because what Maeve and Finn needed as fully blind students and what I needed as a legally blind student at this school were vastly different, especially as my vision worsened throughout my second year attending this prestigious institution. Maeve and Finn had come to the school with all the skills they needed to thrive without sight, but I needed access to learning those skills as my vision and needs changed over time. Unfortunately, it seemed like the school was only willing to accommodate when it was easy and convenient for them. It was as though they were not open to or interested in actually providing the support a student like me required.

During my first year, I excelled. I was in the school musical, **Aladdin**, won a poetry-reading contest, and even received the highest honors for good grades. I was not just meeting their expectations; I was surpassing them. I was popular, making tons of new friends, and for what felt like for the first time ever, not being bullied by anyone. These new friendships extended beyond the classroom. Nearly every weekend you'd see my girlfriends and me in the mall shopping at American Eagle or Hollister; grabbing a Starbucks mint Mocha Chip Frappuccino; or having sleepovers, staying up till 2 A.M. eating Cheetos and laughing at just about anything. No one even seemed to care or judge me for using a cane. It was a relief. It felt like getting a new lease on life. Like maybe, just maybe, I could be my whole self and that was enough.

I first began taking O&M lessons with a white cane when I was in the second grade. I'd be pulled from class to work one-on-one with a specialist who'd teach me techniques to safely and independently navigate the world for that one day when I would inevitably need it.

"Hold the cane centered on your body, around belly button height."

"Run your pointer finger along the flat edge of the handle."

"Every time you step with your left foot, your cane will swing to the right."

Even at this young age in this private setting, I knew this cane made me different. Every time I'd hear that plastic marshmallow shape tip hit the ground, every time I'd feel the pull of the elastic connecting the joints together, I knew I was different. I didn't need anyone to tell me, I knew the rest of my classmates didn't have to experience this. I knew that none of my favorite characters on television were doing this. This made me special. Everyone wants to be special, but not THIS kind of special.

And by the time I was nine that day of "needing it" came. Even though I still felt like I could see just fine, my multiple accidents and injuries indicated otherwise. After running into girls on the soccer field when I was eight years old, I was pulled from playing my favorite sport. And after running into that jagged metal fence a year later, the cane became my unwanted daily companion. To think that a simple fence would be the thing that had changed my life as I knew it... welp—didn't see that one coming!

Once I started using my cane at my old school, the bullying I was already experiencing intensified. Even worse, I was stared at everywhere I went, including by adults. You don't have to see to feel the awkward tension when all eyes are on you. Or hear the way their feet scatter out of the way as if they've seen a cockroach, not a cane. When everybody collectively takes a deep breath and holds it as you walk by, their eyes following your every step, but their movements frozen in time, you know you're the cause. People would make rude comments, whispering their judgments as if I couldn't hear them. Do people not realize that being blind and being deaf aren't the same thing? Needless to say, it was refreshing to feel so accepted at my new school.

A FOUR-LEGGED FRIEND

During the summer between seventh and eighth grade, I went to Quebec to get my first guide dog. After doing a multiday evaluation during spring break, I had been accepted into training at the very place where Maeve got Marble. I'd spend a month living at the guide dog school. Originally the family home of the founder, what was once a farmhouse had since been converted to accommodate blind students and wheelchair users. With multiple dorms, a vet hospital, in-house breeding facility, and kennels, the rural landscapes became a home away from home, despite being much different than the home I was used to. We'd work six to eight hours a day to ensure I'd leave with both a well-behaved dog and all the skills I needed as a new handler. Once I settled in, the matching process began. While most schools pre-match the handler to the service dog before formal training begins, my school takes a different approach. I tested out a male yellow Labrador retriever named Java, followed by a female Black Lab named Cleo, and then finally, a beautiful black-and-white mix of a Lab and a Bernese Mountain Dog (Labernese) named Gypsy! And after careful consideration and a few conversations between the trainers and me, it was decided that I'd get my second choice, Gypsy! And while I originally wanted Cleo, I can confirm they made the right decision.

If Cleo was the calm and quiet one, Gypsy was rambunctious and vibrant. And while I thought I wanted quiet, her vibrance would bring the color back to my life that I would soon no longer see. Gypsy's paws and tail looked like they had been dipped in white paint, and she had a stripe between her eyes and around her snout to match. We were the perfect fit in every way: lifestyle, walking speed, and personality. She was silly, sassy, and full of energy, much like me. I had wanted a guide dog ever since I'd held my first cane. That thing just never felt quite right in my hand. My O&M specialist knew my disdain for this metal stick and promised me that if I worked hard enough on my cane skills, I could get a guide dog when I was thirteen. And that's exactly what I did. From the moment I held the brown leather harness, I knew I'd never go back.

The speed at which I could walk, the confidence it gave me, and the freedom I felt with a dog beside me... nothing could compare. I felt safe with Gypsy, and I knew my parents would likely start allowing me to have a bit more independence with her by my side. The cane had never made me feel normal—the tap-tap-sweeping sound it makes draws that unwanted attention—but Gypsy would draw exactly the type of attention I wanted.

"She's so cute!" I'd hear people exclaim as we passed them on the sidewalk. "What's her name?" "How old is she?" "Can I pet her?" (Questions nobody would ever ask me about my cane.) "Is that a Border Collie?" While these repetitive questions would eventually wear thin, the extrovert in me was so happy to finally have people wanting to talk to me. But the best thing of all? I'd never be alone again now that she was in my life.

I thought bringing a dog to school would make me appear even cooler in the eyes of my peers, and maybe it would have, if I wasn't losing more vision than anyone could have anticipated. At a check-up, the doctors said, "She'll lose most of her vision by her thirties." They couldn't have been more wrong.

While away at my four weeks of guide dog training, I noticed a lot of changes, and in October, my doctor confirmed it. I had lost a significant amount of vision, and there was no way of knowing if it would become stable again. Driving home from that appointment, I felt numb... It just didn't feel real. I knew the signs were there, because I was slowly having to increase the magnification on my computer and struggling more and more to tell my friends apart in their matching forest-green school uniforms. My parents never hid my diagnosis from me, teaching me how to pronounce "retinitis pigmentosa" after school one day when I was in first grade. "Pigman! Pigman!" I'd giggle. I always knew I would one day go blind, I just never imagined that one day was now.

Knowing you'll eventually go blind and actually going blind are two very different things. Perhaps the best way I can explain it (though it is a bit morbid, so prepare yourself) is that we all know our parents will likely die before us, but that doesn't make their death any easier. We don't pre-grieve... There is no way to emotionally prepare for the hole you'll be left with once they're gone or all the ways in which your life will be forever changed by their absence. Just because I was aware this would happen someday doesn't mean I was "ready" for it or ever could be. And let's face it: there's no easy time to go blind, but I'd argue that doing it in the midst of puberty is quite possibly one of the worst. The universe was doing me NO favors.

I went back to school the day after my appointment, and my friends could tell that something wasn't quite right. I wasn't acting like the typical happy-go-lucky girl they were used to. "What's up, Molls, you okay?" The concern in Bailey's voice was obvious. I could make out the silhouettes of my friends surrounding me, their figures contrasting against the light gray concrete of the courtyard. When I told them the news, their reaction wasn't what I expected. I wasn't met with the support, love, hugs, and words of encouragement that I needed, but rather, I was met with a dismissive tone and the words I'll never forget, "Well, at least you're not dying of cancer." Those words foreshadowed the shift in their attitudes that would eventually break me.

What Bailey said was true... I couldn't argue with her, but that harsh sentiment didn't help me feel any better. Someone else's pain did not make mine any less valid, but I couldn't seem to find the words in that moment. And from that day on, my relationship with Bailey and the other girls would never be the same.

I'll never really know why they reacted in such a cold, unkind way. All I can now do is try to give them the compassion they neglected to show me, because they were obviously lacking something in their lives at that time to be so unable to have empathy for others. They may have been going through troubles of their own that I knew nothing about, they may have been jealous of the extra attention I received with Gypsy, they may have just been hormonal teens who were in their self-centered phase, or maybe it was something as simple as poor word choice... I'll probably never know but the reality is, it doesn't matter. What matters is that it happened, and it hurt.

It was more than just drifting apart—I felt like enemy number one. A new girl, Marissa, started at our school and quickly joined our group. She seemed nice at first, talkative, funny, and full of confidence—at least that's what it looked like from the outside. She was sporty, smart, and the girlfriend of one of the cool boys in our class. She immediately clicked with my friend group. Kelsey, Heather, Bailey, Addison, Marissa, and me, we were a classic girl group of besties who always had each other's backs... until like a scene from a teen movie, Marissa seemed to unexpectedly turn sour toward me.

Marissa would make little offhand remarks, taking aim at all my weak spots. She was the queen of backhanded compliments, and sometimes it wasn't even about what she said, but how she said it, that told me everything I needed to know about how she really felt. "Nice hair" never really meant "nice hair" when Marissa was saying it. Before I knew it, she'd turned everyone against me. I was no longer invited to sleepovers on the weekends or to the mall to go shopping. They never talked to me on MSN after school anymore, and I couldn't even try to chat with them on BBM because, unlike them, I didn't have a BlackBerry. Not only could my family not afford one, but BlackBerrys also didn't have screen readers. In fact, no phones did yet, so I couldn't even text them, leaving me feeling so out of the loop. It was so isolating being disconnected from both my peers and society at large, whose inaccessibility was starting to show me that I was invisible. But soon it would go beyond just being excluded from hangouts and being out of the loop on the day-to-day conversations. I'd hear them giggle at me in the hallway or whisper behind my back in class as they'd read the enlarged text off my computer screen, seeing all of my private work. In early February, there would be a grade-wide trip to the capital, Ottawa, and I'd sit alone on the five-hour bus ride.

Headphones on and iPod in hand, I ran my finger around and around the circle, randomly clicking, just hoping I'd land on a song I actually wanted to listen to.[7] I listened to angry music, sad music, downright depressing music, just trying to feel like someone, anyone, knew what I was going through. With my hood up I looked out the window, not for the view, but to hide my face, just praying no one looked my way. Being made to feel invisible made me want to be invisible, something I'd never felt before in my life. Always willing to take center stage and never one to shy away from a little attention, I now wished that everyone else was blind too, just so that they couldn't see the emptiness in my eyes. As tears rolled down my cheeks, I could overhear my former friends in the back of the bus playing truth or dare. They sounded so carefree, having fun the way kids our age should.

The entire trip was miserable and so was I. It was snowy, gray, and cold. Too cold. But I was always cold those days. Too sad to eat much more than a protein bar a day, I was thin, my skin sickly pale, and I was no longer getting a period. Every time I ate, my stomach moaned and my face contorted itself in pain. I felt nauseated a lot of the time, and out of nowhere, my heart would start to race every now and then, but I didn't know why. I hated being in my body, not because I felt fat or ugly or hated anything about it really, but because I just hated being there.

---

7. Apple wouldn't release their screen reader, VoiceOver, on an iPod for another year, so this was my only option.

I'd blast "The Way She Feels" by Between the Trees, or "Like A Knife" by Secondhand Serenade, taking comfort in their sadness. Listening to Hayley Williams belt the words to "Misery Business," I'd belt them along with her. My light, minimal makeup getting darker and heavier, I no longer felt comfortable in the preppy schoolgirl style of my former friends. Classmates started referring to me as an "emo girl"—"emo" being short for "emotional"—and that, I certainly was, and with good reason.

Early on the morning of February 8, we were loading onto the bus to begin the drive back home. This date is notable because it was my fourteenth birthday. The night before, I sat on one of the queen-sized beds in the hotel room that I had been sharing with Addison, Heather, and Kelsey. But now I would tiptoe around them, unsure which version of them I would get. Sometimes we still had moments where we'd burst out laughing about an inside joke from the previous year, when Marissa hadn't yet entered the picture and I could still see the picture. Other times, they'd simply be laughing at me. I clung desperately to the good moments, like little glimmers of hope that I could get back the life I used to have before everything felt so complicated and heavy.

They knew my birthday was the next day, so they decided to throw me a party in the hotel room. We stayed up late past curfew eating my favorite treat, Reese's Pieces, and gossiping about boys. "Jason likes you!" Heather said, poking me in the arm and giggling. My cheeks turned bright red, and Kelsey gasped, "Oh my god! Do you like him back?!"

Honestly, I didn't. I didn't have time to like boys, especially not popular ones like Jason. All the girls liked Jason, including Kelsey, but the rumor that he liked me had been swirling around since last year. I could tell in her tone that Kelsey was a bit jealous at the thought that his feelings might actually be reciprocated, but she had nothing to worry about. Boys were the last thing on my mind; I just wanted to survive.

We continued to laugh and joke around, and it was almost starting to feel like it used to. Marissa was sharing a room with her sister and two other girls from her rugby team, so it was just me and my girls... just like old times. It felt good, and I began to let my guard down, so when Addison suggested they give me a makeover, I didn't give it a second thought. I loved playing with makeup, though it was getting increasingly harder the less and less I could see.

Heather sat behind me in bed and started to style my hair, while Kelsey grabbed her eyeliner and lipstick to start on my face. **Something doesn't feel right.** The coal of the pencil liner tugged its way across my cheek, and they started to snicker. Panicking, I wasn't sure what to do, so I just sat there and let them do what they wanted, acting like I was none the wiser. I pretended to be ignorant and unaware, the way I was learning society expected me to be, now that I could no longer see faces and colors.

UNSEEN

Click, click, click! Flash, flash, flash! I knew Addison was taking pictures of their masterpiece. My hair was sticky with what I thought was mousse but was really whipped cream. And there were words and drawings scrolled across my forehead and cheeks with their makeup. By the next day, the photos would already be all over Facebook and it felt like everyone at school had seen them. Except me.

FAKING IT

My birthday wasn't the first instance my once-upon-a-time friends had done me dirty. It really all began months earlier, at Addison's birthday in November. I was still adjusting to my new reality of rapidly declining vision while juggling how to remain in the good graces of my classmates. ONE YEAR. I'd had ONE YEAR without bullying, and I wasn't ready to give it up and surrender to Marissa and her mean-girl attitude.

At the time, long chains with a pendant that sat just above your belly button were all the rage. While in Addison's basement at the grade-wide party she had, I ran into two of the cool girls as they were exiting the bathroom. Sophie and Hazel weren't in my immediate friend group, but I still knew them pretty well. Knowing how trendy these girls were, I quickly put two and two together when I saw something quite large shining under the lights. I thought it was undoubtedly a necklace. "I like your necklace!" I blurted out, before they walked past me and back out to the party. "Thanks!" I heard Hazel's cute, high-pitched voice call back at me.

Nailed it! I thought to myself. Until thirty minutes later, when I was sitting in the laundry room with a bunch of girls from my class (don't ask—I have no idea why THAT'S where we chose to hang out). We weren't chatting about anything all too interesting when Addison, the birthday girl, walked in with a huff, sitting down next to me. "What's wrong?!" we all asked in concern. "Nothing... they're just talking about one of my friends out there and they aren't being very nice, so I don't wanna hear it." Ugh... I knew. I instantly knew it was me. I shouldn't have even asked, but my shaking voice said, "Who is it?" "Okay, well... I wasn't going to say anything, but... it's you, Molly."

My heart skipped a beat... What could I possibly have done? Turns out Hazel told everyone in the main room that I was faking being blind and she caught me. "She complimented my necklace! She can obviously see."

"I KNEW IT!" Marissa exclaimed.

The rumor began to spread, running wild like an unstoppable forest fire, with my reputation going up in flames.

It wasn't just students who were convinced I could see. Teachers were talking behind my back and to my face. "Molly, help him! He can't see!" one teacher yelled at me in the gym as Finn and I both stood in front of the rock-climbing wall. (Yes, my fancy private school had a rock-climbing wall.)

"Um, I can't either..." I replied, confused as hell. **What does she think my guide dog is for?**

Another staff member, the guidance counselor, even called my therapist to tell her that she thought I was making it all up. I guess it's not that surprising, given this is the same woman who told my parents and me that it was all my fault that I was being bullied because I was being overly dramatic about my vision loss and that I was bringing negative attention to myself.

By trying to use little context cues from the world around me, a skill most blind people have perfected, I had somehow managed to shoot myself in the foot. All the navigation and life skills I had learned as a blind person up until now, in the hopes of allowing myself to be more capable, independent, and accepted by others, had backfired. By trying to mask my blindness and fit in with the sighted world around me, I had seamlessly convinced everyone that I actually wasn't blind at all.

Sometimes it's nice to feel like I can just blend in and go about my day without people realizing that I'm blind, and I know that in many ways, being able to do this is a privilege that not everyone in my community has. It's funny that people accuse me of faking blind, because there are actually times that I fake being sighted.

"Oh, my dog looks just like yours! Here's a picture!"

I'm not sure what people think the harness is for, but... sometimes it's just easier to say, "Yes, I am training this dog," so that I can move on with ordering my coffee and not have to play the Twenty Questions game that usually follows after

I share, "No, this is my guide dog. I'm actually blind," with a stranger. As passionate as I am about advocacy and awareness, making it my entire life's mission and my career, sometimes I do just want to have a normal moment of simply existing as me, the girl behind the disability. But if they've got questions, I've got answers, and I'll take the next half hour out of my busy schedule to talk to them simply because I'd rather they ask and know than assume and be wrong. And if I'm the only blind person they ever meet, I want to give them a good experience that will open their eyes (pun intended) to my community.

However, sometimes I do feel like it would be easier if everyone just immediately knew and understood that my guide dog is there because I am blind. I would love to not have to constantly be the one to speak up and tell people, having to advocate for myself and my needs. And I certainly don't want to have to convince people that, yes, one of the most life-altering things that happened to me—going blind—is real. But unfortunately, I've had to spend a lot of my life trying to "prove" my disability, and it can be even more exhausting than blindness itself. I just want to be able to exist in the world as I am, and for that to be enough. But this wouldn't be the first time I was accused of faking blind, and it wouldn't be the last.

SEEING THE FUTURE

I thought i had hit rock bottom following my fourteenth-birthday disaster, but oh no, I was wrong. The universe has a funny way of knowing exactly what not to do at just the right time. Truthfully, I don't even remember the moment it happened, but somehow I managed to have a classic blind girl accident, something all too frequent when you can't see where you're going. I tripped down the stairs and didn't think much of it but then it started... My ankle ached, it swelled, it was properly injured.

"Brace it and use crutches," the doctor would tell me. "But... how am I supposed to use crutches and my guide dog?" A question I'm certain he had never received before. "Hmm... I'm not sure but I bet you'll figure it out!"

This accident would lead to that fateful day at lunch in the forest that surrounded the school campus. There's no way I could have known then that this traumatic moment would one day be shared with hundreds of thousands of people on stages across the globe. I couldn't have imagined it would spark headlines that would haunt me for years to come, naming me the girl who was "blind and bullied but not broken." Right now, in this moment, that girl is just broken.

That would be the final day I ever stepped foot on those beautiful, historic school grounds. I'd finish the last six weeks of my grade-eight year from home. I felt like I had failed. I wasn't kicked out of school, but I might as well have been. The administration didn't ask me to leave, but they certainly made no attempt to have me stay. The girls who bullied me were never punished; why would they be? Their parents donated large sums of money to the school or sat on the board and mine didn't. I always knew that life wasn't fair, but this was the first time I truly understood the power of money and social politics. If my bullies were going to continue to be enabled and walk through life with silver spoons in their mouths, then I'd rather accept defeat now and go where I was wanted and respected.

I'd spend the summer healing my ankle, and recovering from emergency dental surgery triggered by four impacted wisdom teeth that were living in a mouth far too small for them. In the fall, I'd begin my high school years at a school for the blind, where I could finally start the emotional healing. I would learn all the practical life skills I desperately needed and receive an education in an environment that was built for people like me to succeed. But more than that, it would be a place where I wouldn't be "the blind girl" anymore, I'd just be another blind girl. I, for once, wouldn't be different from those around me. For the first time, I'd get to know what it felt like to live in a world where I was the same as everyone else.

Physically, healing in my high school years looked like a lot of things for me. It looked like changing my diet to heal my irritable bowel syndrome, which had been causing so much stomach pain and discomfort. Eating healthy foods fueled my body and my mind and gave me the energy I needed to rebuild my strength and life again. Mentally, it looked like therapy... and a lot of it. Talking to someone with a total outsider's perspective is a much-needed release. Therapy taught me how to understand myself, process, and work through my emotions in a positive, constructive way. I read self-help books like **You Can Heal Your Life** by Louise Hay, and I leaned into positive self-talk and doing daily affirmations.

Healing was allowing me to find what I was good at again, not just focusing on what I could never, will never, and should never do now that I was blind. Finding passion, something that made me feel alive and valuable, was important. I began to explore new hobbies like singing in an angsty pop punk band, Bury Me Fighting. Music didn't require me to see, so I felt like I was on an equal playing field with my bandmates. And yoga, which inspired me to explore my deeper spirituality. Finding my own spiritual beliefs gave me a sense of hope. I was no longer in this alone; I had someone, or something out there that was guiding me (and not just Gypsy).

I made my first vision board and began working on manifesting the life I wanted. While they may be popular now, they were practically unheard-of at the time. My mom has always been a trendsetter, so when she told me about this concept, I went along with it. I certainly needed her creative flair to help me with the "vision" part of a vision board, so together we sat at the rustic, distressed, dark wood kitchen table and dreamed up a happier future for me. "What do you want your life to be like?" my mom prompted me.

"I don't know..." I responded, finding it difficult to imagine that life would ever get better.

"What about... making new friends!" she brainstormed out loud.

So, I started to slowly make a list of my hopes and desires, while she printed them out and cut up the images. I picked the color of the paper and pen, and she wrote down every word with a smile on her face.

I started small, too afraid to reach for the stars because I had never seen them. I used my mom's suggestion as an easy starting point: make new friends. Pass math class, ace my history final, focus on my mental and physical health, continue therapy, take my supplements and drink enough water every day. But then I started to think, **Why not go big? What do I have to lose? The only thing that can go wrong is that it doesn't happen, and in that case, I'm no worse off than**

when I started. But in the best-case scenario, it DOES happen, and then, well, my dreams come true. So, I went for it. Get a boyfriend and a part-time job. Meet Oprah and be in a Dove commercial! (Very specific, I know, but how else would I find out if these things really work?)

All of this growth and self-development work I was doing was really working. I was not only healing but building a newfound confidence. I reflected on the years of bullying I experienced and realized that I spent so much time trying to fit in and be liked, listening to the popular music, wearing the popular clothes, and trying to be like the popular girls, but... none of it worked, and they bullied me anyway. I wasn't popular, and it didn't make my peers like me, but worst of all, I also didn't like myself. I didn't like that music or those clothes, but I asked myself, **What would happen if I let myself be more true to who I really am inside?**

Away with the preppy-girl style and in with the dark, alternative aesthetic. Gone were the top pop hits, and in were the rock and pop punk. But it wasn't just about changing these surface-level things, it was about no longer living to make others happy. By letting go of seeking the acceptance and approval of others and learning to simply accept myself, I was living more authentically. Now, people were seeing the REAL me, not the knockoff version of someone else that I was pretending to be. Not only did I feel more free and confident within, but that translated into more deep, real connections with the people around me.

UNSEEN

Those manifestations were starting to come true. I was getting healthier; I made new, more genuine friends; and I even got a boyfriend, Jayden. (Remember that band I mentioned being in? He was the guitar player. A classic love story.) And most importantly, I aced that history final I was so worried about! AND even passed math (which has never been my strength). It's safe to say I was pleased with the results of my vision board. It would be my first, but certainly not my last. I was officially a believer.

SHE'S GOING TO BE A STAR!

I wasn't even a year old, just sitting in my mom's lap doing nothing all that remarkable, when Margo, a beloved neighbor and family friend, looked over at me and shrieked, "Oh my god, oh my god, she's going to be a star!"

My mom was rather confused by this unprompted proclamation. "What on earth are you on about now?" she asked, with her warm Irish accent.

"Trust me... I just KNOW that she's going to be famous someday."

As silly as it sounded, my mom trusted that Margo knew what she was talking about. She and her husband, Max, both worked in the entertainment industry, and very successfully at that. Margo was a script supervisor and Max was a cinematographer. They had been on many major television sets and seen many movie stars in action. So, call it an educated guess, call it intuition—or if you're my mom, call it a little bit crazy—but Margo was certain. Little did either of them know at the time that working in Hollywood would one day become my dream.

UNSEEN

After my first big onstage appearance at just five years old, I turned to my parents and declared, "I'm going to move to LA and be an actress!" They chuckled, assuming this was just another one of those childhood fantasies all little girls have, like wanting to be a princess—and that I would let go of this idea and move on to something new eventually. And me becoming an actress felt just as likely as me having a Mia Thermopolis moment (I hope you get the reference). In 1999, seeing a little blind girl on television was as unlikely as the Y2K apocalypse. Diversity? Equity? Inclusion? Nope, never heard of them.

My parents, always wanting to do whatever they could to support me, signed me up for the acting classes that I begged for. Acting class became my escape. I never got bullied there, even though I often tripped and bumped into things because the room was all black, making it hard to navigate with my lack of depth perception. No one laughed or made me feel bad about myself. It was a safe space to let loose and be free of expectations. But the best thing about it was that I got to be whoever I wanted. I was able to take on the personas of characters who were confident, funny, loud, and silly—things that I felt deep down inside but would be ridiculed for expressing outside of those black walls.

These characters I'd play were sighted, and in those moments, I'd get to be sighted too. I might not have been able to actually see, but I learned how to pretend I could. I learned about the importance of nonverbal communication, like facial expression and body language, things that don't always come easily or naturally to people who can't see it. Simple things like looking at someone when they're talking to you aren't necessarily as instinctual as you'd think, especially if you can't see whether you're looking in their direction or not. Small things like waving, sticking your hand out to shake theirs, or nodding along while you listen are concepts that need to be learned when you've never seen them happen in real time. It's almost like a foreign language. When people speak to me using what I call a "visual language"—hand gestures and words like "there, here," or "this," I can't understand it, the way you wouldn't be able to understand Japanese if you're a native English speaker who's never learned it. And while having these skills is useful, in other ways it creates confusion and challenges, and can harm my life and identity.

Thinking it would maybe be another passing phase, like my pottery passion or stint in figure skating, my parents would drive me back and forth to my classes, soon adding dance and vocal lessons to the lineup. I was determined to be a triple threat, just like my childhood idol, Lindsay Lohan.

I first fell in love with Lindsay after watching **The Parent Trap** and trying Oreo cookies with peanut butter (truly a tasty delight!). With the freckles scattered on my nose and cheeks and the red undertones in my brunette hair, I was often told I looked like Lindsay, which was the highest compliment I could have possibly received at the time. My love deepened when I first watched **Mean Girls**, seeing myself in Cady, knowing the hurt of girls like Regina far too well. Forever feeling like the girl who just couldn't seem to fit in, even when I'd tried everything possible to make my peers like me.

After that came my love for Hilary Duff. I'd lock myself in my room singing along to every song on every one of her albums, making up dance numbers for hours on end. I'd watch every episode of **Lizzie McGuire**, perfecting her early 2000s style within my own closet. Blow-drying my hair before school with my leopard-print Stuff by Hilary hair dryer, I'd look up at the posters on my wall and daydream about when that would be me. I'd even had the walls behind those posters painted with the bright pink, orange, and green paints from Hilary Duff's paint line—I was THAT kind of fan.

Each month when my **Seventeen** magazine subscription came in the mail, I'd have my mom read every article and quiz to me. She'd help me cut out images to add to the growing collection of celebrity inspiration on my walls, just like she'd later do when helping make my first vision board.

I loved these girls. They were beautiful, talented, popular, and sighted... They were everything I wanted to be. There was only one problem. I was not beautiful, or at least not in the way the popular girls who bullied me were. They were tall with tanned skin, long dirty blond hair, and straight white teeth. I was short with fair skin and freckles. I had crooked yellow teeth and a crooked eye to match (until I had it surgically corrected). I wore glasses, and none of the boys liked me the way they liked them.

I might be talented, but probably not talented enough for Hollywood to come knocking.

I STILL WON

One weekend in the spring of my ninth-grade year, our home phone rang. My mom answered, and I could overhear her talking to a woman named... Debbie? **Who's Debbie?** I wondered.

Apparently, Debbie read about my advocacy work and fundraising efforts in the **Toronto Star**, and she thought I was beautiful. "Wait, is this, like, a modeling thing or something? Am I being discovered? Like what happened to Justin Bieber?!"

"Well, not quite but close." My mom tried to keep me calm and levelheaded. There was some hesitation in her voice as she went on to explain that Debbie ran the Miss Teen Canada International beauty pageant, and she wanted me to enter as Miss Teen Oakville.

I was excited at the thought that my Hollywood dreams, or something close to them, might be coming true, but I was also hesitant for many reasons. I wasn't even four eleven, a far cry from the typical leggy supermodel girls you see walking the pageant runways. My hair was dyed red and black, and I had an edgy style, not the typical pageant look. Not to mention, the whole blindness thing. I'd never seen a disabled girl win a beauty pageant or even compete in one, so was it even possible?

Jayden (yes, my band boyfriend and I were still together) and my parents encouraged me to go for it. With the three of them supporting me, I decided to climb outside of the box I had trapped myself in for far too long. **I might not win, but I'll still have fun**, I told myself. (But then I still added winning the pageant to my ever-growing vision board!)

As part of the pageant, I'd have to have a charity platform, and I'd also have to fundraise $4,000 and two thousand TEDDY BEARS. Yes, you read that right: two thousand teddy bears donated by the public (technically, stuffed animals of any breed were fine... they didn't have to specifically be bears). The pageant owns a charity, Teddy Bears for Love, that sends stuffed animals to impoverished youth in foreign countries—because THAT'S really what they need. Not food, not clean drinking water, not access to education but a fluffy pink bunny to hold at night. Don't get me wrong, I love sleeping with my toy bunny that my grandma gave me when I was born, but, um... it's certainly not creating world peace. I was still a little naïve though and I was just excited to have a positive project to focus on, so I wasn't going to question it.

Always one to push myself to the limit and overachieve in an attempt to make up for what I perceived myself to lack, I was determined to do THE MOST. I set a personal goal to gather four thousand stuffed animals and $8,000 for Teddy Bears for Love, doubling the pageant requirement. Fundraising for charity was something I'd been doing for most of my life, including recently raising WAY more than $8,000 as a part of my fourteenth-birthday campaign with Ending Blindness, who I chose as my charity platform for the pageant.

    The one thing I knew I was good at and actually enjoyed was public speaking, so that seemed like a good place to start. Together, my mom and I called up local schools to see if they'd have me in to share my story and the mission of Teddy Bears for Love. I'm fairly certain the administrators were more interested in their students learning about vision loss than teddy bears, but either way, I was in! My school allowed me to alter my schedule so I could speak and fundraise. I went to class for two and a half days a week and spent the rest of the time traveling to fundraise. I ended up speaking at what felt like every school in my hometown, including Jayden's. Now I, like Maeve, was on the cover of the town newspaper, and I partnered with the fire department and the YMCA that I worked at to keep the bears and the dollars coming in. We'd have garage sales, bake sales, and every other kind of sale you could think of. We received a donation of fifty adorable hand-knit bears from a local nursing home, and while the money was harder to bring in than the stuffed animals, we managed. Eventually, the basement was filled with a whopping four thousand stuffed animals piled into clear plastic bags, and yes, it was as terrifying as it sounds. I'm pretty sure my parents still have nightmares about it.

By the time the pageant rolled around, I couldn't have been more ready. I took a few weeks off from my job as a camp counselor, packed up my suitcases with all the makeup, heels, and fancy dresses one could want, and headed to the hotel in Toronto where every girl vying for that coveted crown would stay for ten days of festivities. We'd do private interviews with the judges, take an etiquette class (eye roll), perform in a talent show (I belted out "The Climb" by Miley Cyrus), and rehearse for group dance numbers.

Now, I might have been a dancer growing up, even briefly doing it competitively for a year when I was eleven, but it was something I'd long given up. Not even just choreographed dance, but all dance.

At the first dance of the year at my new private school I was twelve years old and dressed as a blue fairy with a body suit and wings to match. I found myself stuck in the middle of the dance floor as "Lips of an Angel" by Hinder began to play over the speakers. One of the popular boys had just whisked Heather away for the slow song. Abandoned, I had no one to help me squeeze through the crowd to the edge of the room where the other singles stood waiting. I was surrounded by slow-dancing couples, loud music, and flashing party lights. I couldn't see, I couldn't hear, and I didn't even have my cane.

I was so mortified. From that day on, I vowed to myself that I would never be caught in that situation again, even if it meant never dancing.

Never dancing, however, was not an option if I wanted to be Miss Teen Canada International! She was a do-it-all girl. She was confident, smart, and funny. Miss Teen Canada International walked, or danced, with a smile on her face and her head held high—while balancing a sparkling crown on top, of course. So, I'd do the only thing I knew how to do. I'd go into "actor Molly" mode. **I'll fake it till I make it,** I told myself.

This version of me was born from years of acting classes and therapy, like a strange coping mechanism I unknowingly developed for times when I felt overwhelmed or underprepared. It had become so easy and natural to turn on this alter ego of mine that I often wasn't even consciously aware that I was doing it—it was a version of me who met everyone else's standards. She was strong, happy, easygoing, and worry-free. It was the me I tapped into anytime I needed to blend in with the crowd, mask my disability, or appear to be keeping it all together, showing no cracks in the face of adversity. I could trust her and rely on her to get through anything. This was one of those moments where she needed to shine.

At our dress rehearsal the day before the big show, a girl would be rushed to the hospital in an ambulance after passing out onstage mid-twirl from exhaustion and dehydration.

She might have had it the worst, but trust me, we were all exhausted, we were all dehydrated, and we were all ready to get this thing done.

And finally, on the day of the pageant, while all the girls crowded around the same mirror, I harnessed all the skills I had learned from watching countless YouTube tutorials and practicing, figuring out my own hacks to do my hair and makeup without a mirror. Counting each stroke of my brush in the blush palette, I'd make sure it was even on both sides. I combed through my straight dyed-red hair, feeling for any strands out of place. I donned the same matching hot pink ruched chiffon dress as the others and stood backstage for our opening dance number, palms sweating, shaking in my gold heels. It was time to shine!

With Jayden and family in the audience, I smiled big and danced my heart out. I might have looked like a fool, but I wasn't going to half-ass anything. I'd already done too much to stop trying now. Before I knew it, I was wearing my glittery ombré pink ball gown with a sash being placed over my shoulder. "Miss Teen Charity," the host announced. I was being recognized for the highest contribution to both my charity platform AND to Teddy Bears for Love. While it wasn't the main prize we were all after, receiving this honor was more than I could have hoped for. Being recognized for all the hard work I'd put in felt like a win for not only me, but for every girl who, like me, had never felt like they could be a pageant queen.

Now they were calling out the names of the top three girls being considered to take home the title. "Miss Teen Ottawa, Laini! Miss Teen Vancouver, Sabina! And Miss Teen Oakville, Molly!"

"Shocked" is an understatement. But I didn't have much time to process. I was being whisked away by a pageant chaperone who took me to a back stairwell, where I nervously awaited my turn to answer one final question that would seal my fate.

Laini went first, then Sabina. We'd answer the same question, but none of us could hear each other through the thick concrete walls of the stairwells. The chaperone gently tapped my shoulder and whispered, "Molly, it's your turn."

Finally! The adrenaline started to course through my veins as I repeated the affirmation **You've got this** in my head. Grabbing Gypsy's harness with my left hand, I took a deep breath, pushed my shoulders back, and smiled as I walked out to the cheering crowd. I heard every click of my heels hitting the stage beneath me and felt the warmth of the spotlight hitting my face as I reached my mark.

The host welcomed me out and then asked, "If you were to win the Miss Teen Canada International pageant, what would you want to be remembered for?" Without even thinking, the words poured out of my mouth like they had been sitting and waiting there for this very question.

"I want to be remembered as the girl who believes that anything and everything is possible. The girl who doesn't take no for an answer and accomplishes anything she sets her mind to. I want to be the girl who never gives up."

I didn't answer the question quite right, not including the exact words of the prompt like we had been taught, but thankfully, that didn't seem to matter. My voice was strong and confident, and my words were clear. I spoke with conviction, convincing myself and everyone else of the truth in those words. This wasn't another one of those times where I'd fake my way through... I meant every word. My answer was more important for me to hear coming from my own lips than it was for anyone else to hear.

After the roars of applause quieted down, Laini and Sabina were invited back to join me onstage. Standing side by side, we grasped onto each other's hands, smiling and whispering nervous "good lucks." I had manifested this very moment on my vision board, but it was hard to take it all in in real time.

"The second runner-up is Miss Teen Ottawa, Laini!" the host's voice bellowed over the speaker system, and I could hardly hear myself think over the sounds of clapping and my own racing heart. Sabina squeezed my hand, and I squeezed back just in time to hear it: "Our runner-up is Miss Teen Vancouver, Sabina!"

More cheers erupted, but they sounded like background noise to my own racing thoughts.

Wait ... does that mean ...

"And this year's winner, Miss Teen Canada International 2010, is our Miss Teen Oakville, Molly Burke!"

As the world somehow both slowed down and sped up around me, I was handed the largest bouquet of flowers I'd ever held. The previous winner placed her crown on my head and a sash around me that was much thicker and nicer than the others. Now wearing multiple sashes and with the weight of a crystal-incrusted silver crown on my head, I looked down at Gypsy, then back up to the audience of screams and flashing cameras. I'd done it.

I'd later find out that while one judge, a well-known reality TV star who had flown in from Los Angeles, hadn't wanted me to win, every other judge had, including her TV star husband. But none of those details mattered to me. It felt like more than winning a silly title or receiving the prize of an academic scholarship and a year of attending fancy events. It was more than receiving validation from a panel of judges saying, **You're good enough!** It was something internal, something inside of me saying, **You don't have to give up and you can accomplish anything you set your mind to. You are good enough, with or without this crown.**

But all good things must come to an end. The joy of the win was short-lived. When we received the pageant contract, my business-savvy dad immediately noticed a million red flags. From the ridiculous ones, like not being able to wear jeans for the next year of my life, to the nonsensical ones, like only receiving my academic scholarship if I went to university within a year of winning even though I was only entering the tenth grade. Suffice to say, I had a lot to consider.

I'm sure not all beauty pageants are as crooked as this one seemed to be. I'm not here to judge the pageant industry or the girls who enter them, because it's not my place, and it feels wrong to do so after having just one sketchy experience with a pageant organizer like Debbie. After many back-and-forth conversations, considerations, and a weird moment where Debbie showed up at my home banging on the doors and windows for us to come outside and give her my sash and crown back, I made the difficult decision to not sign the contract and give up my title to the runner-up, Sabina. I never told the other pageant girls what happened, letting them whisper and speculate as to why Sabina got to live out my reign. Being at the center of rumors and gossip was nothing new to me. Besides, it didn't matter. They could take away my sash, my crown, and my title, but they couldn't take away my win.

I still won.

BLINDBEAUTY07

A year later I started at another new school for grade eleven. Satisfied with everything I had learned at the school for the blind, I was ready to be back at a regular high school, and that's where I met my new friend Brooke. One Friday evening when I was sixteen, I sat on her bed as she applied her makeup. We chatted about our favorite beauty gurus on YouTube, Juicy-Star07 and MacBarbie07 (clearly "07" was good luck, because those girls were crushing it), and all the products they recommended that we were adding to our wish lists. At one point, YouTube had simply been a place to watch music videos or silly cats be silly cats, but now it was so much more than that. After losing my friends and my vision a few years prior, I had stumbled upon videos of different girls talking about all the things that I used to talk to my friends about: dating, makeup, fashion, acne, high school ... I'd watch these girls when I felt lonely, when I knew my ex-best friends were all out shopping together or having those sleepovers without me. I felt comforted by their presence, even if it was only through a screen.

Eventually, they started to feel like they were my friends or even like the big sisters I'd never had.

I'd listen to them do fashion hauls and outfit-of-the-day videos, telling me about the latest trends. I'd listen to them talk about the best spot treatment for those pesky hormonal zits we were all dealing with, or reviews of the latest collection from MAC. They'd tell me about the best pink lipsticks at Sephora for fair skin, or how to do the perfect messy bun. These videos were the new way I was learning how to keep loving all things beauty and fashion now that I could no longer see these very visual trends out in the wild. I couldn't read magazines or see in store windows. I couldn't swatch the colors on the back of my hand to see if they looked all right or scroll Tumblr for inspo. But through these women, I could hear everything I couldn't see.

I'd sit in my room for hours on end practicing, often ending up with too much blush and mascara running down my face after poking my eye with the wand. My parents would lovingly burst out laughing when I'd excitedly run down to show them my work. (They've always been good at keeping me humble, that's for sure!)

My parents have a dry, sarcastic, Irish sense of humor that they bestowed upon me, and it's helped me not to take things too seriously. When I have two choices in life, to laugh or cry, I'd rather laugh, so dark humor has been a big part of my and my family's life. My dad loves making comments like "This blind excuse is getting REALLY old," whenever I ask him to help me find something I've lost, only to have it be found EXACTLY where I was just looking for it (a classic blind girl moment). They'd say, "Blindness is the best thing to ever happen to this family!" anytime we'd score a close parking spot with our disability parking pass or skip the line at a water park. They never felt guilty about passing on a genetic disease, and they had no reason to. They couldn't have possibly known they were carriers of it, and I never felt resentful or blamed them. None of those feelings would do any of us any good. My disability is no one's fault, and acting like it is only turns it into something negative. We've always chosen positivity and laughter in my household... especially if it's about failed attempts at a new hairstyle and outfits that don't match.

Despite all the mistakes, I eventually figured out little tips and tricks that worked for me. I even got so good at doing my makeup and putting together trendy outfits that girls at my new school would ask ME, the blind girl, for help picking out an outfit before a date or the school dance, calling me and describing their options over the phone. They'd stop me in the hallway to ask what eye shadow I had on or where I'd bought my necklace from. To those girls posting beauty videos, I was just another comment or view, and they will never understand the impact they made on my life. They helped me rebuild my confidence and feel less alone. They gave me a space to explore my interests and gain new skills that would translate to making new friends in the real world.

And now, I sat there with this new friend, Brooke, absent-mindedly running my hand back and forth over the seams in her duvet cover. "I think I want to start a YouTube channel one day." Feeling awkward about it, this was the first time I'd shared this idea with someone.

"What would you call your channel?" she replied in a nonchalant tone while flicking her liner into a perfect black wing.

"Mmm... 'Blind Beauty'? I don't know. I haven't really thought about it. Is that stupid?" That was a lie. I had thought about it plenty but just didn't want to admit it. I felt embarrassed—this was well before posting internet videos was considered cool or the job most kids dreamed of because it wasn't even a job yet. I was in my junior year—just one more year of school to go—and I didn't want to give any of my new classmates more reason to make fun of me.

She let out a little snort as she giggled, the same way she always did. "Maybe... I don't know." And that's where we left it.

It wouldn't be until a few months after quitting my job at EAO that I finally felt ready to post my first video on YouTube. I had spent two years of my life opening some of my darkest wounds and sharing them globally. I was, officially, "blind and bullied but not broken," and I wanted to just be Molly again. The girl behind the sensationalized headlines was still inside of me somewhere, but it felt like I had lost her. I wanted to personally explore the parts of me that weren't so connected to my hardships. And I wanted to publicly explore them too. The only aspects of me that society seemed to know about were the ones that separated me from them, which is one of the very reasons I grew up being bullied: my differences, whether real or perceived. Now I wanted to show the very normal, human parts of me. The parts that love makeup, go on dates, do yoga, and collect tea and bath bombs. The parts of me that love to eat sushi, wear pastels, sing along to Taylor Swift, and travel. The parts that connect me to you.

I was so busy while working at EAO that I could only see my friends every couple of months. I didn't have time for hobbies, like downhill skiing, horseback riding, or yoga. Basically, a work/life balance didn't exist, and after almost two years of all work and no play, it was time for me to have a life. In my healing, I knew I needed to find more creative ways to express myself again. I needed to take back the power to share my own story authentically and on my own terms. I wanted the freedom to talk about whatever the hell I wanted to, and most importantly, when I wanted to. I had lost my love for public speaking, the very passion that pulled me through so much pain. I wanted, and needed, to get it back, but it would take time.

While battling my CPTSD, I'd spend my days sitting in my old bed at my parents' house watching the one platform that had always been there for me in times of need: YouTube. I'd search around for whatever content I could find to distract myself from the misery inside my mind. Somehow, I stumbled upon bootlegged episodes of **Shark Tank** and was immediately gripped. Never having been to business school, or even college, I loved learning about and being inspired by these entrepreneurs. These people who would take out a second mortgage on their home because they believed in their baby food brand or quit their six-figure job to pursue their passion for skin care. I saw myself in these strangers, just like I had in the girls posting makeup videos.

I grew up with a strong female entrepreneur in my life: my mom. I had parents who always encouraged me to believe that if all else failed, I could start my own business. "We could open up a boutique!" My mom would get giddy with excitement, thinking up all sorts of ideas anytime I'd get scared thinking about the unemployment statistics I was up against. "What on earth am I going to do for work in a world so discriminatory to people like me?"

"You love fashion! Wouldn't that be so fun?" My parents never pressured me to be anything other than who I am. They believed their job as my parents was to help me be the best version of myself possible, not to mold me into the person they wanted me to be.

So I started to brainstorm what kind of business I would start. Of course I'd offer public speaking, but I wanted to do more. I wanted to sell jewelry and key chains with positive braille messages on them, mugs, T-shirts and tote bags with uplifting quotes I'd write. I could start a charity (one that doesn't suck) to give back to others struggling with similar issues as me. And maybe I could start sharing my life on YouTube.

My parents couldn't have been more stoked to dive into helping me rebuild my life yet again and start my new business venture. They helped me redecorate the guest room into my new bedroom so I'd have a fresh start living back at home. And then we converted my old bedroom into an office so I'd feel motivated to get up every day and go somewhere to work that wasn't my bed, even if it was just one floor below it. I was beyond broke, so they let me live there rent-free and helped me apply for small business grants, as well as loans to help me pay off the medical debt I acquired from Gypsy's sudden and expensive passing. I managed to scrape together enough money to buy an affordable desk, chair, and couch from Ikea for my office, made a new vision board for this next chapter in my journey, and dedicated myself to figuring out how to start and build a business.

I didn't quite know what I was doing but I did know that I never wanted to be at the mercy of someone else again. I never wanted to give my power, control, or autonomy to someone who didn't have my best interests at heart.

"I think I want to start a YouTube channel," I casually mentioned to my parents over dinner one night. "What do you mean?" They both seemed confused by the concept, which confused me. "Like, I want to film videos in my office and post them online," I explained, as if it couldn't have been more obvious. Suddenly, the two most supportive people I knew seemed suspicious and even a little...concerned?

"I don't understand...What is this?"

Okay. I guess I have to spell it out for them. "I want to start a YouTube channel. Like how there's different channels on TV with different shows to watch, YouTube has different channels, and each one is run by an individual person. I want to do that." Silence...just silence. I could feel them staring at me. "Hmm." I could tell my dad was contemplating. "It seems risky. You don't want to be one of those people who embarrasses themselves on the internet," he said, following it up with, "You've had such a successful career as a speaker—you don't want to do anything to jeopardize that." My dad was trading in his typical jovial behavior and dad jokes to put his business hat on.

"Huh? What do you mean? I'm literally just going to be posting videos about things like how I do my makeup or use my phone." I started to feel a bit defensive, like they were judging me for this thing I had wanted to try for so long but had been too scared of, until now. I appreciated that they were just trying to look out for me, but also, I figured I was twenty, I was an adult, and they couldn't stop me, even if I was living under their roof.

SUBSCRIBE

My YouTube channel was by no means an overnight success, but I didn't imagine it would be. My boyfriend of a year, Mark, was the only one supportive of this little plan of mine. Granted, he was also the only person I had the courage to tell other than my parents. He was still attending university at the very school he toured me around a few years prior, and on his summer break he dove into researching the best camera package for me. He drove me to Best Buy, where I purchased a Nikon DSLR that came with a lens, camera bag, and even a tripod—everything I needed! It was a lot of money for me at the time (like, basically all of my money), but I was putting everything I could into becoming a successful entrepreneur, and I was confident that my investment would be worth it one day.

My mom ran her own small business, a gardening company, which she loved just as much as her previous business as a wedding photographer. I needed her guidance when starting up my company, and while she was happy to help with the speaking end of things, she made it clear that other than setting up the camera and hitting record, she didn't want anything to do with my channel. Her gardening schedule worked well with my speaking schedule, with the bulk of my engagements being at schools that were out on summer break during the height of her busy season with gardening. With her help with the speaking portion and Mark's help with the YouTube channel, I felt optimistic that, as scary as quitting EAO had been, I made the right choice.

While Mark was my helping hand behind the scenes, editing all of my videos between studying for midterms and writing essays, he'd also sometimes make little appearances on my channel, including the classic "Boyfriend Tag."[8] His college roommates, who also happened to be his best friends, were the first to find out about my YouTube channel when they saw Mark helping me film a dog toy haul while I was staying with them—and unfortunately they were quick to make a mockery of it.

They invited their girlfriends over and Mark and I could overhear them playing our Boyfriend Tag video on the big-screen TV in their living room, all the while laughing at us, knowing we could hear them from his bedroom.

It felt like a punch to the gut. **THIS is exactly why I'd been hiding my channel from everyone!** My stomach was tied in

---

8. A popular video trend where couples film themselves answering the same list of generic relationship-related questions—how did you meet, favorite drink, birthday, and so on—so the audience could learn about your partner and you could see how well your partner knows you.

knots, filling with shame while I heard their mocking voices call out to us, "Oh my god, this is so funny!" It wasn't funny, actually. And neither is making fun of someone for following their dreams, especially when you're supposed to be an adult. Even though I knew they weren't trying to be malicious with their remarks, it still hurt. I felt like I was in middle school again, being bullied and having to hide my true self. I hadn't had the confidence to stand up for myself back then, but I did now.

I could tell Mark was embarrassed. "This is fucked up," I said, heated. I thought I was past this point in my life. With a rush of emotions coursing through me, I charged into the living room, looked directly at them, and before I had time to think, I opened my mouth. "Are you serious right now? Do you think you're being cool? Do you really think that it's cool to be laughing and making fun of people you're supposed to be friends with? You're in your twenties and you're acting like children. Grow the fuck up and stop behaving like high school bullies. I'm doing something I enjoy, Mark is supporting me like a good partner, and you're just sitting there on the couch doing nothing productive with your lives. Are you proud of yourselves? And you know what? Someday I'll be really successful, and you'll look back at this and be so embarrassed, filled with the same shame you're trying to fill me with."

Okay, I admit it, I might have gone a little TOO hard on them. But it certainly did shut them right up. Laughter turned to awkward silence, the TV was turned off, and as I walked back to Mark's room with my head held high, he met me halfway and gave me a hug. "I'm sorry," he whispered. But he had nothing to be sorry for. Shaking in his arms, my body still filled with adrenaline, I could hear them calling out their apologies from the other room. The apologies were nice, but I didn't need them. The feeling of empowerment that washed over me as I began to calm down was the only thing I truly needed from this.

In many ways, this moment was healing. It healed the inner child who couldn't fight back against the mean voices. The one who'd let those mean voices win and control her. The one changing every piece of herself to fit their narrative. She'd become uncomfortable in her own skin to make others more comfortable around her. That girl was gone and had been replaced with someone who knew her worth, felt valuable, and had a strong sense of self. I now had a spirit that couldn't be so easily broken, and that spirit would carry me through the next few bumpy years as I navigated growing a business and creating content. And while this wasn't the way I'd wanted the people in my life to find out about my channel or the reaction I'd hoped for when they did, their negativity didn't dissuade me. In fact, it made me feel more passionate than ever. They were the people I needed, the people to prove wrong.

In those early days I was hardly getting any views, which made their comments sting even more. While the disability community is thriving on social media now, it certainly wasn't back then. The YouTube algorithm worked on recommendations—if you watched a makeup video by one beauty guru, it recommended you another makeup video by a different beauty guru. With there being almost no openly disabled creators making content, none of my videos would be pushed into people's feeds. It felt nearly impossible to be discovered by new eyes. It was a vicious cycle, and while some may have given up and focused all of their energy on more lucrative endeavors, I kept posting my weekly videos.

Worst-case scenario, it was just a fun, creative hobby, and best case, it was a marketing tool for my motivational speaking business. Either way, I didn't care because it was something enjoyable to focus on outside of my daily fears and stressors. I trusted that eventually the right people, or even one person, who needed my content would find it. It could make a difference in some small way or another. Plus, it was a great way for me to stay connected to the audiences at my speaking engagements. The middle and high school students I'd speak to were basically the only people watching my videos anyway. I'd try to plug my channel at conferences and events whenever I could: "I'm less than a hundred subscribers away from hitting a thousand!" I mentioned casually during the Q&A at the end of my speech, and that night, I hit that 1K milestone.

Even though my social media career wasn't exactly taking off, in other ways my business was thriving. I was not only taking on more and more speaking clients, but I also began hosting two weekly television shows that aired nationally across

Canada, sharing interesting stories about all things disability and accessibility. My first year in business, I managed to break even, a huge win for me! I even earned the exact same salary that I'd had at EAO while working a fraction of the time. Can't beat it! That was truly all I could ask for.

I might still be pretty broke, but at least I'm happier.

A SQUEAKY-CLEAN CALL

I hopped off the plane at LAX with a dream and my guide dog, Gallop (and yes, I was singing the iconic Miley Cyrus song while doing so). It was 2016 and I'd flown in from Toronto to speak at VidCon on a panel about online accessibility, something I was very familiar with as a disabled woman and (maybe up-and-coming?) content creator. As a relatively small YouTuber with only five thousand subscribers, I still couldn't believe I was there surrounded by social media's most popular creators of the 2010s and some of the very people who inspired me to post my first video. iJustine, Rosanna Pansino, Joey Graceffa... I was surrounded by internet royalty. The buzz of the weekend ahead was palpable. I clutched my coveted yellow badge, the only one you can't buy because it's reserved for the Featured Creators and VIPs. **I might just be one step closer to making my dream a reality.**

Given my slow start on social media, I never expected YouTube to be my career, or to randomly receive an email almost two years into posting weekly edutainment and lifestyle videos.

YOU'RE INVITED! read the title, and it continued: **Hi there! I'm Lauren from VidCon and I'd like to invite you to speak on a panel at VidCon 2016 in Anaheim, California . . .**

As I read on, I thought it must be a mistake, a joke? Maybe even a scam? **There's no way this is real and actually meant for me.** But, sure enough, it was.

Eight months before this monumental email popped into my inbox, my two-and-a-half-year relationship with Mark ended. This, however, did not stop my mom from suggesting boldly, "Maybe Mark should be your plus-one to VidCon!" (They'd always loved Mark, and for good reason—he was a great guy, just not my forever person. So, ummm, no, Mom, I don't think so.)

Convincing my mom to come with me was just as hard as convincing her that Mark shouldn't. I knew I needed her; there was just no way I'd be able to do it on my own. The anxiety of it aside, navigating an unfamiliar environment with the crowds, all the loud noises, the packed schedule of speaking on three panels, plus meetings and parties . . . it wasn't going to happen. My mom accompanied me on all of my work trips and speaking engagements, so I didn't understand why this would be any different. But to her, it was. Even though I would be speaking at a conference, something I did all the time with her by my side, my mom viewed my YouTube channel as being separate from my work, not a part of it. Thankfully, she eventually gave in, even though she was certain Mark and I would have had more fun.

In preparation for my first VidCon, I bought a few trendy, new "Instagrammable" outfits, even though I wasn't even on Instagram yet, having no one to take my photo. I even had my mom study the faces and names of all the other Featured Creators so that if she saw one of my favorites, she could guide me over to them so I could introduce myself. I packed up business cards and attached colorful braille key chains I'd had made on Etsy with my name engraved on the back (one of the many products I'd gotten custom made in the hopes of starting an online boutique). I wanted to be memorable to all these new people I was sure to meet, and this felt like the perfect way to stand out from the crowd.

Once we arrived, we spent all our free time in the fancy branded lounges only available to Featured Creators with access via that VIP yellow badge. We'd snack on the little finger foods and people watch (to clarify, she'd people watch... I'd people listen), striking up conversations with whoever happened to sit down nearby. We're both outgoing, so this came naturally!

On our final day, a nice man took a seat on the couch next to us, clearly tired (but hey, we all were). Neither of us had any idea who he was, but we'll talk to a brick wall if it's the only thing around, so... "How's your VidCon going?" my mom asked. He rambled off an answer about how wonderful but stressful it is each year, then returned the question.

"Well, I'll be honest. I didn't really know what to expect and wasn't really looking forward to coming, but it's just so incredible! The impact these creators are having on people's lives... They're so vulnerable and honest, it's refreshing!" I couldn't believe what I was hearing come out of my mom's mouth. Then she turned to me. "I really think we should focus on YouTube more! You could really do this. It would be a great way for you to connect with people around the world and share your message, but you wouldn't have to travel as much and risk getting burnt out on the road again!" Ding, ding, ding! She was getting it!

Something else pretty special happened that weekend. Sitting in yet another fancy, exclusive, creator-only lounge sponsored by Facebook (now Meta), I jumped on a Skype call with a casting director. I had been taking calls with her and her team for a "secret beauty brand" project for MONTHS at this point and STILL didn't know what these special "auditions" (literally just me chatting with some women and answering their questions) were really all about. But I was finally going to find out.

It all started with an email popping into my business account asking if I'd be open to speaking with a casting agency for an undisclosed "major brand" opportunity. On the first call, they admitted that they themselves weren't quite sure where this was going. "We're meeting with a bunch of different women and just kind of . . . seeing what jumps out at us. For example, we've met with an artist, a new mom, a marathon runner, and now you. We can't say much about what we're working on yet, but we thought a blind person could add a unique perspective, so we'd just like to chat and get to know you a bit and we'll take it from there."

A few Skype calls later, and I had convinced them! Of blindness being a cool angle, not of me. "We love the blindness thing, and we were wondering if you have any other blind girlfriends who you think would be open to chatting with us."

In this moment I had to decide what was more important to me: the opportunity for ME to be a part of a major beauty campaign or the opportunity for a blind woman to be a part of one. I knew it was a great chance to increase authentic representation, whether it was with me or with someone else in my community. So, as much as I wanted it to be me, the answer was obvious. "Yes, I have tons of them! I'll ask around and let you know who's interested!" I managed to wrangle ten or so of my most beautiful, charismatic, charming, and fun blind besties to audition. Some I had known for nearly as long as I could remember; others had come into my life in more recent years, whether it be from summer camps, retreat programs, or the school for the blind. It's a small community, so when you build a connection, you keep it, even if you only keep up through social media, because many of us don't have people we can truly relate to in our day-to-day lives. I loved these girls, but it was hard knowing that my friends were also now my competition going into the next round of auditions.

I was at the picnic-in-the-park-themed lounge at VidCon, which was the only place that had a strong enough Wi-Fi signal for me to be able to take my final call—a stressor in itself! I sat at a wooden table, rubbing the bottoms of my shoes back and forth along the fake grass beneath them.

"Well, we can finally tell you the name of the brand." I could hear the smile on the casting director's face as I tried to block out the background noise of all the creators networking. "The commercial is for a new body wash from Dove."

The vision board was still doing its damn thing, all these years later. If that's not proof that manifestation really works, then I don't know what is!

NO ROOM FOR A GIRL LIKE ME, HUH?

In August I'd shoot the global print and commercial campaign for Dove Shower Foam. And so would one of my best friends, Dani, who I met at a summer camp for the blind when we were both eleven. We'd swim in the freezing-cold lake together and she'd jokingly splash me and laugh at my squeals of dismay because I HATE cold water. We'd sit beside each other at every meal, her making fun of me for always spilling my water and grabbing my freshly washed hair with her sticky maple syrup covered hands just to get a rise out of me. Dani was a tomboy, and I was a girly girl. We didn't get along at first, but eventually we grew to appreciate our differences and, even more so, our similarities. We'd stay up eating Skittles and talking all night, just happy to have someone who understood what it was like to be both in the sixth grade and legally blind. And we'd now have another thing in common because Dove ended up casting both of us, but "only one of you will get the final spot that airs on TV." **Is this my first real introduction to the cutthroat world of entertainment?**

They explained to us that we'd both film the same commercial and take the same images. Because Dove doesn't script any of their ads and only works with "real women," they liked to cast two or three people for each campaign. "Some women freeze up on camera, or don't give us the sound bites we're looking for." They had already prepped me for the fact that "we won't be giving you any specific direction or prompts because we want it to be real and authentic, so we like to have options ... just in case one doesn't work out the way we're hoping." I even had to sign a legal document verifying that they didn't give me a script of any kind and didn't instruct me on what to say on camera.

Three grueling twelve-hour shoot days in the boiling hot, humid summer heat, and Dani and I were done. I had shot my first commercial, but would it even be seen by anyone? It was hard for me to fully enjoy those three days on set. It was surreal being surrounded by hundreds of crew members and big professional trailers with free food, getting my hair and makeup done, working with a stylist ... but while I was in the spotlight, I found myself constantly comparing myself to Dani. **Am I as pretty as her? Is she funnier than I am? She's so smart and talented, and everybody loves her.**

For Dani, shooting this campaign was a cool experience. Something fun to look back on in twenty years and tell your kids about. She was an artist, a behind-the-scenes creative with aspirations of being an event planner or designing displays in store windows. But for me, this was not only a career opportunity, but the chance to live out young Molly's dreams, and I didn't want to let her down.

In the months that followed the Dove shoot, I tried my best to put it out of my mind. Worrying about it wouldn't change the outcome. I needed to focus on things that were within my control, like YouTube.

"We need to find you a manager!" My mom eagerly shared this grand idea with me as we drove from my parents' house in the suburbs into downtown Toronto. We were attending an event at the YouTube Space, a creative hub for Canadian YouTubers to gather, network, and film content. Since attending VidCon in June, I had managed to grow my modest five thousand subscribers to twelve thousand, and while that still wasn't impressive to the room of creators I was walking into, I felt really proud of having accomplished this in just four short months. But . . . "I'm not big enough for a manager!" I brushed off my mom's silly suggestion before unbuckling my seat belt and stepping out into the crisp fall air.

Sometimes moms really do know best, though. That night I met the man who is still my manager to this day. Following a presentation from a YouTube exec, I asked a question during the audience Q&A, and it caught the attention of some fellow creators. They approached me during the mix-and-mingle hour with their manager Reuven in tow. While I spoke with these creators, whose best advice for me to keep growing was to "go viral" (**Gee, thanks! I hadn't thought of that one yet**), he and my mom got chatting. She somehow convinced him to set up a one-on-one meeting for later that week. When we had our first coffee, I was instantly drawn in by his infectious energy. I'd never met someone who was so sure of themselves. Everything from his style to the words he used was just so utterly Reuven. I already knew he was somebody special, and after six months of "dating," we made it official and I signed on as his newest creator.

Even when told by industry experts that "there's no room in the business for someone like her—don't bother," he believed in me. "Just wait, she'll be my biggest creator one day," he'd tell the skeptics.

Well, yeah, there's no room in the industry right NOW, but that's what I'm here to change, I thought to myself after Reuven shared the closed-minded, ableist things he was hearing about me. Sipping coffee at yet another trendy café Reuven suggested, we'd brainstorm all the ways to grow our businesses. He was just as new to the world of social media management as I was to the world of content creation. We were in it together, but it would be an uphill battle, and Reuven wouldn't always go easy on me. But I was prepared for the industry and the critiques that came with it. I had a thick skin. So when Reuven gave me some pretty brutally honest tough love, I didn't take it personally. I trusted that it was for my greater good and if I worked hard enough it would benefit both of us.

"What are some dream brands you want to work with?" Reuven asked. Dove had been top of the list for so long, but I checked that off once finding out that my commercial had been the one selected to air globally. My voice was dubbed over in multiple different languages, and my foamy shower photos (they were tasteful, I swear) would be plastered on billboards and cardboard cutouts in Shoppers, CVS, and Walgreens across North America. Now with that completed, I knew who was next. "Aerie!" I confidently told Reuven. "I want to be one of their #AerieREAL Role Models one day!"

Similar to Dove's commitment to using unscripted "real women" and real stories in their advertisements, #AerieREAL Role Models were unedited and unfiltered in every way. Aerie worked with strong, empowered women who stood for something, like Olympic gymnast and outspoken sexual abuse survivor Aly Raisman, and body positive "plus-sized" model and mental health advocate Iskra Lawrence. They showed stretch marks, acne scars, lumps, and bumps in all of their authentic, beautiful glory. These women weren't pretending to be perfect on their billboards; they were loving and accepting that they weren't. Aerie's values as a brand aligned with all of my own values. It helped that I also genuinely LOVED their comfy, stretchy clothes and colorful, unique swimwear. I was a fan of the brand **and** a fan of the branding. I wanted to be a part of all of it.

THE GUY WITH THE GLASSES

For almost two more years I'd been upgrading my filming setup, collaborating with other creators, and experimenting with different styles of content. Making space in the industry where there was none was a big undertaking, but I'd been making headway. I was ready to pack up my life (and favorite Anthropologie dishware) into seven suitcases and finally make the move to LA. This move wasn't just the result of my social media career, it was the completion of that childhood dream of living and working in Hollywood. But in order to actually move to America, I had to be successful enough to prove my value and qualify for an O-1 visa, otherwise known as the visa for "individuals of extraordinary ability," which was NOT an easy task. But finally, I'd done it and was legally allowed to live and work in the United States. Which had me asking myself, **Is this it? Have I made it?** Ah, how naïve that girl was.

The idea of "making it," well, I just don't know if I believe it really exists. My life has been a series of peaks and valleys, which is what it's like for most people but especially true when your career hinges on a computer algorithm that doesn't care about you as a human being. Years of therapy and plenty of hardship in my teens and early twenties taught me that you have to learn to live for the ups and ride out the downs, knowing the upswing will eventually come again. The downs are hard, but they're also where you learn the most important lessons. Growth isn't easy, but it is rewarding. The next stage of my life and career brought with it many of those hard but important lessons and helped me grow into the woman I'm proud to be today.

I was spending my nights sleeping on a hard, cheap mattress on the floor while spending my days running to TJ Maxx and Marshalls to pick up whatever cute but affordable home decor I could find to bring my girly, glittery, dream apartment to life. Okay...maybe not a DREAM apartment. More like an outdated one-bedroom with vertical slat blinds that reminded me of sitting in a doctor's office in the '90s: dreary, dark-brown cabinets, and a sun-bleached, cream carpet. But it's what I could afford for my first LA apartment, and I'd make the best of what I had.

My mom came along (on her O-2 visa—the partner visa to my O-1) and planned to spend the first two months helping me settle in before heading back to Canada. One day nearing that two-month mark we received a phone call from my dad, the man behind the business bills, making sure all of my corporate finances were in order, taxes were filed, credit cards were paid off, and my mom and I got our monthly paycheck.

(Basically, he took on all of the business-related tasks I didn't want to. Thanks, Dad!)

"You're running out of money." I heard the stress, almost panic, in his voice. "You might have to take out a loan, or I don't know how you'll make rent." Now I was panicking too.

Ever since I'd gotten my first job at fifteen, I had been paying for anything that wasn't a necessity. If I wanted a grande unsweetened matcha latte with soy milk (no foam) from Starbucks or to go see a movie with my friends? I would pay. If I wanted a pair of limited-edition, multicolored Ray-Bans or some buttery soft Lululemon leggings, I would pay for them. Socks? Toothpaste? Advil? My parents would still cover the essentials. Until I was eighteen and moved out: then ALL the bills were on me. Fair enough! I liked paying for my own things. It made me feel independent in a way that I really valued, and I valued everything I purchased because I WORKED for that pair of sunglasses (that I still have to this day, fifteen years later). But as hard as I worked to buy nice things for myself and as much as I tried to save up, I had spent years draining my bank account trying to grow my business. I'd invest the little I was making back into it, leaving me without much wiggle room.

I've been fortunate enough to never have to take on much more debt than a credit card bill from the cost of Gypsy's passing, which was paid off within a few months. I didn't have much, but I had always managed to get by. **I just don't know how on earth I'm going to make this work.** I couldn't disappoint that five-year-old girl who so proudly said, "I'm going to move to LA!" She had finally done it, so I had to figure this out.

Walking down the sidewalk with Gallop calmly guiding me on my left and my mom on my right, I chatted with her.

"The building across the street looks really nice! Very modern, clean, bright... big windows." She described the surroundings to me as we went, the same way she always does.

"I'll live there soon enough!" I proclaimed, manifesting my way out of this financial hardship I had found myself in. Vision boards, manifestation, thinking positively, living with gratitude: these were the only tools I had to keep me afloat when times got tough. They'd worked before, and they'd work their magic again!

On my birthday I received a package at my door. "It's a present from the team at Samsung!" my mom told me. I had recently begun building a relationship with them following an introduction from Casey Neistat, who had taken me under his wing just six months prior when I was stuck at sixty-four thousand subscribers.[9]

On the final day of my second VidCon, my mom started loudly whispering to me, "Molly! It's that guy! The one with the glasses!" She knew her role—see for me! Spot all the creators I'd love to meet. But...

---

[9]. Turned out that nice man we had spoken with was one of the bigwigs at VidCon, and he had taken a liking to my mom and me, scoring me another invite.

"Who's the creator with the glasses? Lots of creators wear glasses." I had no idea who she was talking about.

"You know, that cool guy! You know, he does those airplane videos and lives in New York City!"

"Casey Neistat?!" I exclaimed, a little louder than I should have.

"YES?" he said, standing right next to me, turning around to look over his shoulder when—"A dog!"—he spotted Gallop and immediately dropped to the floor for pets and cuddles. **No, you aren't supposed to pet a guide dog when they're working but who cares, it's Casey Neistat!**

I took my "in" while I had it and knelt down next to him. "Oh my god. Hi, I'm Molly. Sorry, I had no idea you were there, I'm actually blind and this is my guide dog..." Not knowing how long I had with him, I quickly pitched him on a video idea I knew he couldn't do without me. This meant that if he liked the idea, he'd HAVE to collaborate with me... a method that had worked well for me in the past. Sell them on you, what sets you apart... a reason they need to work with you or your business over any other.

To my delight, he gave me his email. "Let me know if you're ever in New York City. I'd love to film with you!"

Like any sane person would do, I emailed Casey and told him that, "I actually have an upcoming girls' trip to New York!" It was a total lie, but hey, he said to let him know when I'd be in New York, so... I had to find a reason to be there! I didn't want to look like I was so desperate to film with him that I was going to fly there JUST for that (even though I was)—your girl can hustle. Once our collaboration went live and I was seen by his over eight MILLION subscribers, I was catapulted into the 100K club overnight (subscribers, not money—I was still broke).[10]

Casey's belief in me couldn't have come at a better time, as I'd been experiencing a total standstill in my growth for months (channel growth... my physical growth peaked around eleven—thanks, genetics!), and I was quickly running out of money. Thanks to Casey and my budding relationship with the marketing team at Samsung, I had grown enough of a following and made enough money to move to LA, but now I wasn't sure how long I'd be able to stay if something more didn't change. Bad luck for me, because this was the peak of the YouTube "adpocalypse," where, following a horrific and harmful viral video from one of the largest creators on the platform, brands started to pull their ads to avoid being associated with potentially negative content that wasn't seen as "brand friendly." Videos were being demonetized, and it would take months (if not a year or two) before YouTube would regroup and sort out how to both protect advertisers and pay creators fairly again. So I, along with all creators, wasn't making nearly as much

---

10. In fact, I had forgotten my bra when I traveled to NYC and was filming in a white shirt, so I ran to a Victoria's Secret and purchased a bra to wear for filming and then had to return it... SHHH!.

through ad revenue as people would probably assume by looking at my views.

Opening the birthday gift from Samsung, I took a deep inhale as a warm, woody aroma filled the air. I picked up a heavy jar, feeling smooth wax and a wick inside.

"It's beautiful!" My mom described it: "The glass is clear, and the candle is white with a white label. Let me read it." I passed it to her. "Le Labo, Santal 26." She passed it back to me, and I took another deep breath before placing it on my coffee table. That scent became the symbol of hope for me, because shortly after receiving the gift I also received a job offer from them. I was going to be in a Samsung commercial that would play at the Oscars, and with that paycheck, I'd manage to keep paying rent loan-free. That job saved my ass, and from then on, every time I'd fear the future, I'd smell that candle and tell myself, **Everything will be okay**.

IF THE SHOE DOESN'T FIT

In no time, I was breaking the lease on my crappy little apartment and moving into that modern, bright, clean one just a few blocks down. I chose a two-bedroom because my mom had been sleeping on the pull-out couch in the living room for far too long. (Thankfully, she loves sleeping on couches, for some unknown reason.) Two months came and went, and my parents and I collectively realized that my career was getting bigger and busier faster than we could have expected. I needed my mom not because she was my mom but because she was my assistant, and like anyone in my position, I needed an assistant, and there was no time to hire and train someone new. That didn't stop us from trying, though.

I met up with a follower who sent me a message on Instagram a week after I moved into my first LA apartment. Risky? Maybe, but I was desperate to settle in, make friends, and build connections with locals who could show me the ropes. Luke's message was warm and inviting, and he wanted to take me out for coffee to welcome me to town. He was SoCal born and raised, a cool, sporty, and artsy guy, all things I liked.

There were some things we didn't quite connect over, though. Unlike me, Luke was conservative and churchgoing. But hey, I'm open-minded, and maybe a spiritual community would be the warm and accepting group I was looking for. Turned out the church was also where Justin Bieber and Selena Gomez attended, among many other industry elites. Yes, I was really in Hollywood!

Despite the fact that I had little to nothing in common with this church community, it was all I had in those early days. Without them, I'd have no one, so I found myself trying to force friendships that weren't meant to be. It was like shoving my foot into a shoe that was a half size too small, thinking, "It's SO CUTE! And on sale! I can make it work." No, girl, you can't. After ten minutes of walking in those things, you'll want to rip your feet off—we know this. But it somehow felt better to have someone, even if it was the wrong someone, than it would be to have no one, especially once my mom left town.

Eventually, after some trial and error, flaky fake friends, and dating a few losers and users, I found my people. If there's one thing about LA that I love (aside from the weather, of course!), it's the creatives who live here and celebrate individuality and self-expression, and allow you to be whoever the hell you want to be, without judgment. THOSE are my kind of people!

Moving to LA allowed me to feel like I could start fresh. Back home, it felt like everyone knew who I was and what I had been through and I was stuck being that person in their minds forever. It held me back and made me feel like I was stuck being that person too. In LA, I was no longer that "blind and bullied but not broken" girl. Instead, I was this interesting, outgoing, cool content creator. I was adult me, not fourteen-year-old me, or eighteen-year-old me. People were meeting Molly, the real girl behind the story. In fact, they didn't even know the story, and I loved it. It felt freeing and gave me permission to explore who I was and find the right people who connected with that person.

Before finding that group, though, I made the mistake of moving Luke into the second bedroom of my new apartment and letting him live rent-free (plus a small paycheck) in exchange for taking over from my mom and becoming my part-time assistant. This would include attending meetings and events with me when needed, taking my Instagram photos, filming my YouTube videos, and other random tasks while still giving him time to pursue his own work.

He had a professional camera, lights, and all the talent needed to help me produce my content and would be just a door knock away from helping with any at-home emergencies. My mom and dad would be reunited in Canada, and I could be the big, grown-up girl I was ready to be again. All was well. Just kidding... Nothing was well, **especially** not me.

My mom's bags were packed and ready to go, and it was perfect timing, because I'd booked a gig back home in Toronto. I flew with a week's worth of stuff, and her with everything she owned. Two of us flew there, but only one would return to LA.

After spending a week in my old bedroom at my parents' house and being in the cold, snowy March weather, I was ready to get back to sunshine, palm trees, and my new roommate, Luke! Although he would actually be away for the first few days, so I'd be completely on my own (well, Gallop would be there, but you know what I mean). It was no big deal, though; I'd lived on my own before. "A few days will be fine," I assured my parents.

But then, what's that? A tickle in my throat? A blocked left nostril? The day of my big flight I woke up feeling like death. I arrived at the airport bleary-eyed with a pocket full of tissues and cough drops... not how I'd planned to spend my first few days of freedom.

I thought my dad would be the biggest fan of my mom moving back home with him, but instead, he was the biggest naysayer: "She needs you. Her business needs you." I overheard him on a call with my mom, encouraging her to stay as she packed up to leave.

"I can always come back. Molly wants this; she's ready." She's always had my back! Needless to say, he was surprised and a little dismayed to see her come home with so much luggage in tow.

"What's all this for?" he asked as we rolled up to the front door of my childhood home.

"I told you, I'm moving back," she replied.

When I woke up sick, he encouraged her once more to return to LA to be with me. "Just bring your passport with you, at least," he urged.

"Don't be silly!" she said, swatting at his arm as we walked out to the car. Turns out, sometimes dads are right, and she should have brought the passport.

After checking in at the ticket desk, I turned and gave my mom a snotty, tearful goodbye. "Everything is going to be okay," she whispered. "I know ... I just wish I wasn't feeling so sick," I told her. I continued to cry the entire way through security and customs. The tears just flowed uncontrollably, which I hadn't expected. The airport staff member who was guiding me to the gate didn't seem to notice, or maybe she just didn't care, but the border guard sure did. "Secondary," he said, handing back my passport. "Follow me."

I was escorted off to a small room, where I'd wait to be questioned further about my US work visa and ... my tears? I couldn't use my cell, but it wasn't long before my name was called. After questioning, I was approved to fly, and while walking to my gate, I checked my phone to see my mom had called. Phoning her back, I heard the ring, ring, ring, before she finally picked up. "You called?" I asked.

"Yes, I'm coming! Your dad brought my passport, and I'm just going through security now! I'll be on the flight!" And just like that, the tears dried up in relief.

Waking up the next morning, I could barely pick my head off the pillow and couldn't even bear to open my eyes. A splitting headache, snot-filled sinuses, and a sky-high fever? Yep—I was sick, and I was so happy to have my mom. In the days that followed, I was sicker than I had been in years, and without my mom there to take my guide dog to the bathroom and spoon-feed me cold, soothing yogurt so I could take my meds, I don't know what I would have done.

Luke didn't last long before I felt forced to let him go and ask him to leave the apartment. Breaking nearly every rule I set for him, including regularly bringing a girl over who openly bullied and made fun of me, missing deadlines, and lying to me all proved that he couldn't be trusted. The last thing I wanted was to live and work with someone I couldn't trust. I guess even churchgoing good guys can be bad boys behind closed doors. Luke was out, and my mom was back in, and that was how it was going to stay.

AMERICA'S NEXT TOP ROLE MODEL

With my mom by my side, in the coming years, I'd have many new apartments and hair transformations, walk countless red carpets, board hundreds of flights, work with nearly every major creator and partner with numerous dream brands, including Aerie by American Eagle.

That's right, my manifestations worked once again! At first, Aerie contacted me to do a simple, one-off Instagram post for their new bra. But then they reached out with the offer of a lifetime. I got the call while sitting at the hair salon with a head full of pink dye. "They want to sign you for a one-year contract."

Stunned, eyes wide, mouth open, I looked like a real-life shock-faced emoji. "Are . . . are you serious? Is this real life?" I could hardly contain my excitement, heart racing, doing silent squeals while Reuven kept going over the offer on the other end of the phone.

"I don't care what it is, just take it, I'm in!" I rushed to say in a concerned tone, as he began to raise issues about some of the points in the deal.

"You deserve more than they're offering for this much work."

Reuven was used to brands lowballing me, hearing things like, "Our disability budget is lower." **From a brand who wanted me to promote how inclusive they were for blind people.**[11] Or, "If we put her on a billboard, no one will know she's disabled." Aka **We won't get brownie points with the public for being inclusive because she doesn't look like a minority.** Reuven was a fierce believer in me, my talent, and what I deserved, even when I wasn't. "I don't care, this is a dream come true, I'll take it," I replied.

"No, let me see what I can do," he responded confidently.

"Okay, but just... don't fight too hard, I don't want to lose this opportunity." It's a phrase I've frequently used with him, but thankfully, he rarely listens and always wins.

I might not be able to see, but my love of fashion has been around since well before I could even dress myself. I come from a long line of fashion lovers, including my grandma, who designed and handmade wedding dresses. As a toddler, my mom would stick me in a stroller when I'd get fussy and walk me around our local mall, knowing that looking in the store windows would soothe me. I still have a binder filled with all the drawings of outfits I dreamed up; I even took sewing classes and made my own pajamas. I'd beg my mom to bring her professional camera into the backyard to do mini photo shoots with me. My parents even booked me a professional

---

11. I'm hoping you see the irony here without me having to spell it out.

studio shoot when I had to start using a cane so they could create something fun out of such a traumatic event. I put on all my best outfits and posed, cane in hand, against the white backdrop. Standing under those studio lights, I felt like I was exactly who I was supposed to be.

The first time I remember ever seeing representation in media was while watching **America's Next Top Model**. (Obviously one of my favorite shows as a fashion-loving girl with superstar ambitions.) It was 2004, the very same year I became a full-time cane user. I'm of course talking about Amanda from Cycle 3. Partway through the season, she was faced with a big obstacle. That week's challenge was not just any runway walk, it was a nighttime one. Fine for most people, but not if you have retinitis pigmentosa, like Amanda. She opened up and shared that she is night-blind (the first major RP symptom). It's safe to say I was rooting for Amanda to win and was crushed the day she was voted off.

It's hard to understand the need for representation when you've always had it. I never had it, until Amanda. It's hard to believe you can accomplish something when you've never seen someone do it. Seeing Amanda on my television screen made me feel like I could do it; watching her and her talent get overlooked by the judges hurt me on a deeper level than just watching a reality contestant lose the competition. But I never forgot about her.

Now, with Aerie, I could be someone else's Amanda. This was more than a paycheck to me—this was paying it forward. I didn't have to worry about the paycheck, though, because Reuven worked his magic, as he always does, and I got what he knew I was worth. I signed the contract, and I was officially an #AerieREAL Role Model. My photo would be in store windows, in email blasts, on the website, and even on billboards. I wasn't just an "influencer" now: I was a REAL model and ready to inspire other young girls the way I once needed to be inspired by someone.

DUMBO

My days at EAO lacked support and control but with my new career, I called the shots. I decided what was worth it and when. I had the autonomy my therapist had once insisted I needed. I knew at any point I could choose to push pause and take a step back, or even give it all up, and knowing that was enough to help me keep my head above water. I knew it wouldn't be like this forever and I had to soak up every moment while I had it. Plus, the opportunities I was getting, like a ten-day European adventure courtesy of Samsung to celebrate reaching a decade of blindness, were far better than going to rural middle of nowhere Iowa to speak to a hundred people. (No offense, Iowa.)

Frankly, a lot of those years are a blur at this point. If I wasn't working, I was sleeping. I'd board the plane, sit in my seat, 2A, and nap before the flight from LA to New York had even taken off. I'd wake up upon landing, climb into another big black SUV sent from a car service, and fall back to sleep as soon as I arrived at the hotel. This level of exhaustion was worth it, and I loved every moment I was awake.

I'd pinch myself. **Is this real?** I was in constant awe of my reality.

Suddenly, I was getting these opportunities I had watched my favorite creators receive, never imagining it would one day be me. With my mom on my left, Gallop at my feet, and Emma Chamberlain on my right (NBD), our early morning Delta flight took us from LAX to JFK once again. We'd pack a lot into just one week. First, we'd be in Brooklyn for the Top Creators Summit, a multiday event hosted by YouTube. They rented out an entire hotel for the top one hundred creators. Listening to speakers like Kris Jenner by day, drinking cocktails and listening to live music by night... I felt like YouTube royalty. (If only Mark's old roommates could see me now—oh, wait, they can... all over the internet!) **I have to commemorate this once-in-a-lifetime experience.** And as if the universe had read my mind, I opened an email forwarded by my management:

We noticed Molly is in New York!

The email came from a well-known tattoo magazine, and they were wondering if I'd be open to appearing in a video on their social media where I'd do a "tattoo tour," showing off and explaining the stories behind my tattoos. I'd grown up watching both **Miami Ink** and **LA Ink** on TLC. I had loved body art ever since. After getting that first tattoo with Rebecca at just seventeen, I racked up an additional four more. I had been toying with the idea of getting a new tattoo to celebrate my internet achievements, and who better to do it with than this magazine that had access to all the best artists in New York? "I'd love to!" I replied before pitching my idea.

"I'd also love to make a video for my channel, if you're open to it!" I explained. "I want to have my followers vote on a tattoo idea and then get it WITHOUT knowing what it is!" This felt like the ultimate way to honor my followers, the only reason I was getting to have so many mind-blowing experiences to begin with. I'd show them how much I trusted them, that I was willing to get a permanent piece of body art based solely on their choosing. And to my delight, the magazine agreed to provide an artist and camera crew for the next day. **Well, no time to think, no time to change my mind, we're in it now!**

I quickly updated my followers, posting an Instagram story and a Twitter poll. On one platform, I gave them the choice to vote between a black-and-white or colorful piece. On the other platform, they could select between four tattoo ideas: an elephant (my favorite animal), a grapefruit (my favorite fruit), a glass of lemonade (because I like to think I've spent my life turning lemons into lemonade), and a palm tree (to symbolize my LA journey). The vote was open, and the appointment was booked. In the morning I'd be off to film a collaboration with Doctor Mike (perhaps the internet's most famous medical doctor), where we'd play the nostalgic board game Operation and I'd get to ask him all of my most burning medical questions (like the one about my toenail fungus—fun!) and then on to get some fresh ink!

I'll admit, I was exhausted, running on just a few hours of sleep. I had laryngitis from too many days of socializing and was a tad bit hungover following the final party of the summit. Despite that, Doctor Mike and I filmed two successful videos (one for each of our channels) and it was now the moment of truth... What would my new tattoo be?

At this point I was so busy I had not one, but two assistants. My mom and Lisa. Lisa had been working with us part-time for a number of months and joined us midway through this hectic trip to lend a helping hand. A bit overwhelmed and wanting to prep for the next New York adventure, Lisa attended the tattoo session with me while my mom packed up our hotel and relocated us to the next one in Times Square. Divide and conquer was the only way to get it all done.

Lisa and I walked into the tattoo shop and were immediately struck by the uncomfortable energy. The video crew was running late, and everyone seemed to be confused as to why we were here. We sat and took a second to catch our breath. The nerves hit. **Is this a bad idea?** But Lisa assured me, "Your mom and I will look at the art before she tattoos it, we'll make sure it looks good, don't worry!" Famous last words.

The team finally arrived, but the energy still felt really... off. I overheard the producer and videographer make snippy remarks back and forth. There was an air of stress around everyone. They were so distracted by their own negativity, it was like they were ignoring us. I should have seen the red flags, but... I'm blind, so can you blame me for missing them?

"All right, what are we doing?" the cameraman blurted out.

I explained my concept before asking, "Do you want to film your video first or mine?" The tattoo artist then walked over and introduced herself. And action! I guess we were starting with mine...

"I think they probably went with elephant." I told her how well my followers know me. "I'm always like, 'I love elephants.'"

She laughed.

"If it is an elephant, and they chose color..." I continued. Given I had purple hair and was never one to shy away from a little color, I had a strong feeling that's where the vote would land. "I love a lot of my tattoos to be just black outlines, so maybe to include color... do pink ears and a pink tip of the nose." I nervously shared my vision for each option with the artist so she had a few guidelines to work with. "Just don't make it look like Dumbo!" I insisted while on a break between filming. I covered my face with my hands and cringed. I knew by not choosing to approve of the design, I was giving her a certain level of creative freedom, but I was hoping she would still take my parameters seriously.

My mom, Lisa, and I had all agreed that Lisa would text an image of the design to my mom before I got it tattooed. I could only assume Lisa forgot in the midst of all the chaos, because she solely approved of the design without my mom's valuable input. While this was likely an honest mistake, my mom's eyes are the ones I trust the most, so this was a big deal.[12]

"Why are you getting an elephant? What does the elephant mean to you?" the cameraman asked me partway through the tattoo. A silence fell over the group as if in collective shock at his misstep. With the sound of nothing but the tattoo machine buzzing, I glared daggers at him, and in a cool, icy tone I responded, "Well, I guess I'm getting an elephant, then, huh?"

"It's rolling, right, you're rolling," the producer jumped in.

"No, I cut," the cameraman said as if it was not a big deal.

Of course, the camera isn't rolling. With the big reveal ruined and half the tattoo still left to go, I didn't know what to do, but I was too tired to get worked up about it. I was pissed off, there was no turning back the clock and unhearing what he'd just said. I had to think on my feet and figure out how I was going to save this video that meant so much to me and my followers.

Lisa used her sharp tongue and made a snappy remark at him, but he brushed it off. "It's not a big deal; just pretend you don't know when we reveal it on camera at the end." His apathy was infuriating: he didn't understand how monumental this was to me. I've never faked, pretended, or lied to my

---

12. Having to rely on others about my appearance will never get easier.

audience about anything. I'm always an open book, almost to a fault. Admittedly, sharing everything comes more easily to me than creating healthy boundaries of separation and privacy with my community online. I didn't want to fake the reveal, but I also didn't know how to tell the truth in front of a group of people encouraging me not to. I didn't want to disappoint my followers, who were eagerly awaiting the tattoo reveal vlog—I could be disappointed that the surprise was ruined, but I didn't want to disappoint them.

"A little baby elephant! I knew it!!" I feigned surprise as the soapy bubbles were wiped away and the tattoo was revealed on camera. But not to worry: there was one surprise still in store. The elephant was in color just as I predicted. However, my wishes were not respected when it came to the design. I found out it was larger than I'd anticipated, and it was filled in with a 2010s galaxy-print design akin to something you'd find on tacky leggings. The whole body had clouds of pink, purple, and blue with twinkling white stars inside. Well, color me SHOCKED! "I would never have thought of that!" I said, attempting to use a cheery voice, employing "actor Molly" once again to avoid hurting the artist's feelings.

The experience was ruined, the vibes were bad, the tattoo was not what I'd wanted, and now I had to show the one person I trusted to be brutally honest with me...and I knew she wasn't going to like it. She knew me, my taste, and my style better than anyone.

Lisa could tell I wasn't happy. "It's cute! I'm sure your mom will love it!" she encouraged me in the taxi on the way to our new hotel. Unfortunately, she was wrong.

"Oh... wow... um... it's Dumbo?"

UGH, not the response I was hoping for. She didn't like it, and I wasn't so thrilled either. I wasn't honest in my video about the surprise being revealed, but I figured I could at least be honest about my thoughts on the final result.

At the end of the day, art is subjective. Just like my videos, or even this book, not everyone will like it, and as a creative, I accept that, even if it hurts sometimes. I sat on it for a bit, thought things through, and gave the tattoo time to heal, but when I arrived home to LA and finally released the video, my honesty was not well received. My audience was hurt that I didn't like what they had chosen for me, and the artist was very offended, even though many of her own fans said that they didn't think it was her best work. She began to send threatening messages to my team, and I found myself in my first-ever internet controversy. Being a longtime people pleaser, this was really hard for me. I tried to decide whether I should stand up for myself, or give in, delete the video, and move on as if it never happened. (Not that that was really possible, given I had a permanent reminder of it on my left arm.)

Ultimately, I'd chosen not to approve of the design before having it permanently placed on my body, which was fully on me, and I had accepted the consequences of that choice. But what was harder to handle was upsetting both my audience and the artist. So, keeping the video up felt like more stress than it was worth. Even though it felt like the artist hadn't listened to my design request, which had hurt me, I still didn't want to be the one responsible for hurting her. Years of being on the receiving end of pain at the hands of others had made me hypersensitive to the idea of being the cause of that pain in someone else's life. **My life has been filled with enough drama. I don't need to make more for myself**. I decided to take down the video. Now I no longer had a special piece of content to honor my followers and the success they afforded me, and I had nothing but a negative memory attached to this damn galaxy elephant.

Even worse (okay, not WORSE, but maybe just as bad?), the magazine ended up editing the footage that was filmed for my channel and posting it on theirs. We never filmed the agreed upon "tattoo tour" that was supposed to be for their channel. It struck me as extremely unprofessional and felt like it had all been for nothing. I considered starting laser tattoo removal but found out that based on the colors incorporated, it would take years and might never fully come off. I decided to let go of my frustration and bad memories and try to focus on the original intention behind it: my followers. I figured one day I'd alter it slightly as a way to create new memories while maintaining its existing form.

UNSEEN

Five years later, while on a business trip in Texas, I had some free time and decided to be just as spontaneous as I was when I got that now-infamous elephant (you know, since it worked out SO well for me the first time). Googling "tattoo shops in Houston," I found one with good ratings that accepted walk-ins, and finally added a quote that makes the piece feel complete. "Sky's the limit," it reads, next to the starry elephant as he gazes upward. Today I have a permanent reminder of some of the craziest years of my life AND of the phrase my parents raised me on that allowed me to get here. Sky's the limit, baby! And don't forget it... you never know where that belief might lead you.

"SHORTY" GIRL PROBLEMS

That New York trip was a memorable one for more reasons than just that. It seems the theme of the trip was... spoiled surprises? The final day was to be another one of those **pinch me** moments at the Shorty Awards. (Think the Oscars or the Grammys of the social media world.)

I had gone from attending award shows to being nominated for them. I was up for Best in Lifestyle at the Shorty Awards against girls I loved, creators I looked up to and who were everything I never felt like I was. Working in such a visual industry without sight, I felt like I couldn't possibly live up to the content of the other nominees. But there was one thing I was confident I was good at: public speaking.

On top of being nominated for an award, I was asked to present one. As I sat in the hotel room with my freshly bandaged tattoo, I read through their script so I could practice. "And here to present the Shorty Award for Best in Hospitality, Shorty Award winner Molly Burke!" **Um, excuse me... WINNER?** Yes, they sent me the wrong script. It was hard to feel excited when I was so exhausted and disheartened by the day's events: two big surprises ruined in one day. I couldn't feel much joy in that moment knowing that what should've been a big celebration, with the sounds of cheers and congratulations, had been stolen by a script that should never have been sent to me. It was very anticlimactic. I found out about my first big industry win while sitting on the edge of my hotel bed as the robotic voice of my screen reader droned on.

But while I wouldn't be surprised by the win at the award show itself, I was still surprised that I had won at all and hoped I could share in that enjoyment when I was well rested and dolled up the next day.

I was sitting at a round table dressed in an extravagant Oscar de la Renta gown in the front row of the venue. Red lipstick on, I could see the bright stage lights just a few feet away. My category was introduced, and I sat calmly, waiting to hear my name, but then... **Wait! What if the script was wrong?** My heart started to pound with every word the presenter said.

"Oh my gosh, this is one of my favorites! And the Shorty Award... Ah, I'm so excited to announce this one! Okay, the Shorty Award goes to... Molly Burke!"

Sigh. What a relief! I quickly stood up in my red high heels, grabbed Gallop's harness in one hand and Reuven's elbow in the other. As the crowd cheered around us, he guided me up the steep stairs to the podium where I delivered my acceptance speech. I purposely hadn't written one, wanting to keep the authenticity of a real surprise.

"Ah, oh my god, okay... I'm very overwhelmed. First off, shout-out to everyone else in my category: you're all amazing and inspire me, so I'm kind of shook that I'm the one up here. Also, huge thanks to my amazing manager, Reuven, and the rest of my team..." I continued on with the typical acceptance speech, thanking family, my followers, and of course, Gallop. And then something really important came to me: "It's quite ironic that I'm winning Lifestyle because I'm someone who, as a blind woman, lives a very unique lifestyle. And as someone who grew up dreaming of being in the entertainment industry as an actress and a model, when I went blind almost eleven years ago, I never expected that I'd get to work in this industry still. And along the way, there've been so many people who told me that I wouldn't, and I can't, and I shouldn't, and there was no place for me here. So I just want to say that if you're disabled, if you've been bullied, if you live with mental illness and you want to work in this industry and you feel like there's no place for you... there is. Keep going, because I'm living proof that you do deserve to be here."

And in that moment, I felt like maybe I did really deserve to be there. I'd continue to battle imposter syndrome, and it's hard not to when you're literally the only openly disabled person in every room you walk into. But I was finally starting to feel like I was gaining the respect of the industry.

Getting dressed up and going to all these fancy events in flashy ballrooms alongside the very creators I grew up watching felt unreal. It was amazing and a dream come true, but on the other hand...something felt wrong. I was the only "out" and visibly disabled person there. While my channel had grown significantly, there were still few disabled creators, and none seemed to be breaking into the mainstream creator space like I had somehow managed to. The pressure I felt to represent my community and do right by them was immense. But every time I'd be faced with inaccessibility or ableism, I didn't feel I had the power to speak up because I was simply "lucky to be there." I was constantly battling the same thought over and over again: "Do I really deserve to be here? And if so, why me?"

PRETTY GIRLS WALK LIKE THIS

I was in all the right rooms, collaborating with the best brands and the biggest social media stars. From the outside, life once again looked pretty perfect. And I'll be honest, in many ways it felt that way too—more than ever before, my dreams had come true. But one dream still remained. I might have been at the parties and filming with the "cool kids" of YouTube, but what I really wanted was to actually be one of the cool kids of YouTube, something I still didn't feel I had accomplished. I wanted to be friends with them, not just their internet friend who they would hug and say hi to at the next PR party, or take a photo together for Instagram, but the real friend who they'd text for advice or simply to hang out outside of "working hours."

A lot of my followers found me through these big collaborations I was doing, or would be excited to see me film with one of their favorite creators. They would assume, based on our positive online chemistry or those photos they'd see of us together, that we were really friends. I'd go live on Instagram and people would ask, **How is XYZ creator doing?** and I'd dance around it, finding a way to answer the question without admitting that we weren't REALLY friends. "Oh, I love him too! I don't know... he's good... He's been super busy lately, so we don't really talk much outside of events and stuff." All true, but I was failing to admit that the reality was, we didn't talk outside of events because we weren't real friends, we were just friendly with each other. Even though I often wanted to be friends.

I didn't want to ruin the illusion for our followers, and I was embarrassed to think that I was interesting enough to collaborate with but maybe not interesting enough to hang out with.

Our collaborations were mutually beneficial business transactions, and I got as much out of being "the blind girl" in their video titles as I got out of having their name in mine. Viewers seemed to be more upset about me being called "the blind girl" than I was. I understood my role in their content, and at the end of the day, a title is how you market the video to potential viewers; it's what makes it clickable. I was virtually unknown when I first started doing these collabs, so putting my name in the title would mean nothing to anyone outside of my small subscriber base. I'm grateful for the opportunities I had to be on these big platforms that reached more people than I ever could have on my own. They got a unique video idea and lots of views by having me on their channel, and I got a greater chance to educate and increase representation. But that doesn't mean my own insecurities didn't rear their ugly little heads from time to time. The creators I collaborated with were all nothing but lovely, supportive, and kind toward me, so I tried not to take any of it personally when they didn't text me back or invite me to their Christmas parties. **They really are super busy! They're probably workaholics like me. They have enough friends. They're like this with all the other creators too.** And in many cases I'm sure a lot of that is true. But it was still hard feeling like the world was seeing me as this popular, cool, blind internet girl, and really inside I was still battling many of the same demons I had while trying to navigate social relationships when I was growing up. I still craved the feeling of "fitting in" and was doing what I felt I had to in an attempt to finally achieve that.

I found myself decorating my apartment in the same generic gold, gray, and millennial-pink way that every lifestyle girlie on Instagram did. White faux-fur accents, velvet tufted couch, and a touch of tacky bling. I'd pose in front of the iconic angel wings on Melrose and the famous pink wall with a pink drink in hand (even though I never liked the pink drink). I would shop at the cool boutiques they'd all haul in their stories and use the same filters on my feed. I found myself once again losing me to become one of them.

Them—the pretty girls, the cool girls, the successful girls. The girls who I wanted to be like and be liked by. I wanted to be their friend, to live their life, to finally feel accepted by my peers in some weird, subconscious attempt to heal my inner bullied child. Even though I'd earned the right to be there just as much as anyone else, I still didn't feel like I truly belonged. I wasn't really like them and never would be, but I couldn't let them know that.

Hindsight is 20/20 (even for me). I know now that I was dimming my own light. I was neglecting to see that my success was because of my uniqueness, not my sameness. The more genuine I became, the easier it was to make real, strong connections. I was finally starting to show up as the fullest version of Molly. Sometimes you have to learn the same lesson twice before it sticks.

I spent money I shouldn't have to buy the Cartier Love bracelet that we were all supposed to wear to show we've "made it," and the double-G Gucci belt because that's what you did when you were a young, hot influencer... you got influenced by all the other influencers who told you how to be on trend and stay relevant.[13] I felt an added internal pressure to do and buy these things because I constantly felt the need to prove to myself and others that I was successful despite my disability and against all the odds. I wanted to be the opposite of everything society expected of me as a blind woman. They think I can't work? I'll make so much money I can buy a $7,000 bracelet. That bracelet would serve as a subtle signal to the world that I am more than you think I am capable of

---

13. Though, admittedly, I do still wear that bracelet AND I do love the Gucci "GG" logo because my first two guide dogs were Gypsy and Gallop, so it kind of felt like it had its own little special meaning just for me!

being. I should be taken seriously and finally viewed as equal in this industry and in life.

I wanted to be everything no one had expected of me. Everything I'd long feared I would never achieve. Spending that money on a designer item on Rodeo Drive while still renting an apartment felt like a terrifying risk, but one that I needed to take. I was far from one of those young wealthy influencers who were so easily willing to blow thousands, if not hundreds of thousands, on fancy things and a bougie lifestyle.

I worried if I did it would all disappear overnight. I'd be the "one-hit wonder" of social media, and this ONE brand deal or ONE successful month would be a flash in the pan, and I'd never experience this level of income again. So for a long time, I continued to spend and live the same frugal way I did when I was broke and struggling to pay bills. Even if this meant I was limiting my own comfort, happiness, and even my own potential. I wouldn't make investments in my own career, like buying props for content or hiring a more qualified editor or better assistant. Even though these things could have possibly delivered a big return, I felt like I was making money that might have to last me a lifetime.

Seeing this pattern, my dad began to hop on a monthly finance call with me. He'd go over my expenses for the month, how much I'd earned and spent, and what was in the bank. We'd discuss what brand deals or speeches were upcoming, and what payments were still pending from previous work. I learned that if I feared money, I'm attracting that energy, but if I trusted that the universe will always provide, it will. Buying those items felt like breaking free from my self-doubt. From then on, it became easier to loosen up and slowly let myself spend the money I was working so hard to earn (within reason, of course).

I was wrapped up in a fast-paced world of views, numbers, clicks, and titles, all while navigating being a disabled twenty-something in a new city, growing a career, running a business, making friends, and (unfortunately) even swiping on Tinder. And doing so with the world watching (and sometimes judging) me online.

HATERS GONNA HATE

During the first few years of posting on social media I was accused of faking my blindness (isn't it funny how history always seems to repeat itself?). I was very clearly faking because "she's looking at the camera!" or "her eyes are blue not milky gray"[14] or a classic, "she's not wearing dark sunglasses." And so many other nonsensical stereotypes that stem from the portrayal of blindness in mainstream media. But this isn't mainstream media, this is real life, and I am a real blind person, not a sighted person playing one. I would receive comments saying that I was "faking it for clout" (because apparently disability clout is a thing? Wish I had known that growing up!) or "social media fame," even though my content was hardly getting any traction.

---

14. This stems from the stereotype that all blind people's eyes have a specific appearance to them that can come from conditions like cataracts (something that I do not have). This is perpetuated by mainstream media, which often has actors who are playing a blind character use blind sclera contact lenses that cover both the iris and the sclera and change the look of the eye.

Once my channel did start to grow, the comments would say I was "only successful because I'm blind," despite the fact that at that point, there still were no big blind or disabled creators and being blind had actually made it harder for me to grow my channel. I was struggling to get my content into the recommendations, having naysayers in the industry, and seemingly getting demonetized if I used the words like "blind" or "disabled" at one point, thanks to YouTube's old ad filters. (Apparently, disability wasn't ad-friendly?)

So which one is it? Am I only successful because I'm blind, or am I successful in spite of the fact that I am? This question would whirl around my mind, flip-flopping depending on which answer suited my imposter syndrome better at the time.

The reality is, someone like me had never been successful in the industry, so those naysayers didn't see how it was possible. Thankfully, I always choose to take the path of most resistance because the reward was SO worth the fight to get it. I chose to let negativity fuel my fire, making it burn bigger and brighter than ever before. I choose to see every "can't," "won't," and "shouldn't" thrown my way as a dare. And I'd always take the dare. You couldn't tell me no, because I'd just say, "Watch me." And watch me they did.

Every time I received a hate comment, I'd remind myself I was one view closer to my goal and their comment only served to help my engagement (a very important metric in the social media world). Every ignorant comment I read would ignite my passion to keep going, keep educating, keep expanding people's minds, and keep representing people like me.

The sense of responsibility to do my community justice never left me. The lack of representation and the misrepresentation in mainstream media has been deeply damaging to the disability community. I personally hold the belief that the majority (if not all) of the continued oppression and discrimination against disabled people comes down to the way the media has historically depicted our stories.

The disability community is still the least represented minority in all media, and the majority of the time our characters are written, directed, and played by non-disabled actors who cannot and do not represent us with the authenticity and accuracy we deserve. This only furthers the stereotypes and misconceptions that make our daily lives even more difficult than they already are. The media is often the only access many people have to learn about disability, making it that much more crucial for it to show our true lived experiences.

Growing up I never saw a Victoria's Secret model in a wheelchair in store windows or an inter-abled relationship on TV. There wasn't an amputee mother taking care of her child on the big screen or a neurodivergent lawyer being depicted. When you're never seeing these things, disabled people, especially women, are not viewed as valuable or capable, contributing members of society. We aren't viewed as beautiful, sexy, desirable, smart, funny, talented, or even human. This leads to us being quickly and easily dismissed when we apply for a job, swipe right on a dating app, or simply try to live a normal life. When the media portray disabled people as nothing more than disabled, reliant on others, and "different from," it only furthers the divide that already exists between us and you.

Many people were raised being told, "Don't point," "Don't stare!" and being shushed when they dared ask a question about a disabled person. The truth is, kids don't do these things to be rude or mean, they do them because they are curious and want to learn about the world around them and things they are unfamiliar with. With children's media having the least disability representation among all forms of media, the only way they really learn is from looking and from asking. So many generations are now unlearning the fear of disability that was built for them as young children. The same fear that now leads them to want to avoid disabled people rather than interact with them because they've never been taught what to say or what to do. They don't realize they simply need to treat us as they would any other human being because we've been dehumanized by society and the media for so long.

YOU CAN'T BUY EQUALITY

I used to daydream about when I'd be successful enough that my disability no longer mattered. I'd walk into any room, heads would turn, and my guide dog or cane would have nothing to do with it. People wouldn't awkwardly fumble over their words when striking up conversation because they were nervous they'd say the wrong thing and offend me, like, "You're so pretty for a blind girl!" but because they were so excited to meet their favorite celeb.

You hear that money can't buy happiness, and I've learned that success can't buy equality. No amount of internet followers, magazine articles, or even money can help me buy my way into a more equitable world. This realization slapped me in the face while my mom and I were standing in the cool night air on a sidewalk in Studio City outside of my friend's apartment. It was March, and we'd just spent the evening sitting on the couch, sipping red wine and having fistfuls of popcorn as we watched the Oscars. Not for the stars, but for the commercials.

until I left the establishment, shaking with a mixture of anger, fear, and humiliation.

On my twenty-ninth birthday, I was unable to get a ride to my favorite sushi restaurant. And years before, I was on the way to the studio to record my audiobook, **It's Not What It Looks Like**, when the driver, angry that I was in his car with Gallop, began filming me while speeding and driving erratically, yelling at me and threatening to call the cops (a great way to start such a big day!). And we can't forget about the gem "Fuck my dick!" as I tried to explain that, yes, my guide dog is to me what a wheelchair is to someone who can't walk. I've been told, "You're not blind, you fake-ass bitch." Classy! You'll be getting five stars from me!

Being brought to a festival in Central Park by a major medical brand didn't stop me from being caught in a stampede with ten thousand people charging toward me after fears of an open shooter broke out. Being put up at a fancy hotel by a major tech brand didn't stop the doorman from telling me, "The rooftop is full," and yet ... two minutes later when my non-disabled manager walked up to the same doorman, suddenly there was space available. Being Molly Burke didn't stop the bouncer at a club from telling me to "get to the back of the line." No matter how much I told him, "I'm on the VIP list ... I'm literally being paid to be at this event tonight." But when Casey Neistat walked up and told him, "She's with me," oh, sure, then he could suddenly find my name on the list.

I get it... I'm not the person people expect to see in these spaces. A little disabled girl isn't who you think is deserving of these opportunities, and that's exactly why I'm there. I like to turn heads; I like to stand out and be exactly what people don't think I should be. But even with that, I've learned over the years of growing my career that no amount of public status or high-powered friends, and not even that Cartier Love bracelet, removes injustice or discrimination. It doesn't make the world more accessible or accommodating; it doesn't remove all of the barriers and hardships that disability can cause on a daily basis. After years of facing it head-on, I now find myself going into fight, flight, freeze, or fawn every time someone tries to deny me access, wondering, **Will it be another enraged bartender or rude driver? Will I be put in an unsafe position at this event? Will they have even thought of my needs? Do they care to?**

Don't get me wrong, my career has brought with it many privileges, and I recognize that. I'm grateful to now get a car service to bring me to my interview, speaking engagement, or onto set. But it's not because I'm bougie or fancy (well, not JUST because of that); I don't get things like this for the same reason other people in my industry do. I get it because when my client is paying me to show up and do my job, I can't risk being put in the wrong frame of mind by having to fight for my rights, cancel, and call another ride. As hard as the realization is that I'll never be successful enough to no longer feel disabled by the world around me, I'm also glad I can't buy my way out of discrimination or oppression because it keeps me fighting for every disabled person who isn't in these rooms and doesn't have these opportunities. And if nothing else, damn, does it keep me humble.

One thing that gives me so much hope, though, is that I no longer feel I am in it alone. A rare gift the pandemic brought us was the rise of TikTok, which ignited my career in new ways. But more than that, it helped shine a bigger spotlight on disabled creators, and the presence of the disability community on social media increased at a rapid rate. There is now a thriving community of disabled creators sharing their lives, their creativity, and their talents with the world. Educating, raising awareness, and normalizing disability in a way we've never seen before. Finally, my community is receiving opportunities that are long overdue. They are running successful businesses while changing society's perception of us. I couldn't be more proud and happy to see where we are today. Social media has allowed us to have greater autonomy and take back our power. Sharing the past decade of my life online and making all of those growing-up-in-your-twenties mistakes for the world to judge hasn't always been easy, but I tell ya, every time I meet another disabled influencer who says, "You were the first disabled creator I watched, and you're the reason I started. You made me believe I could do it too," THAT... that right there makes it all worth it.

LAST NAME BURKE

Aside from social media, I'm happy to report that I am seeing a slow but notable difference in mainstream media. I'm increasingly hopeful that the media industry as a whole is trying to move the needle forward on inclusivity and authentic representation. I think that the increased social media representation and the clear interest shown by the general public in disability-related content has pushed mainstream media to step up and do better by us. In the past month alone I've watched five NEW disability-related films, some even hitting "select" theatres. Some documentaries, some scripted indies, but all showcasing real experiences of disability. All the hard work of countless disabled advocates and creatives may finally be paying off, and it's a long time coming. But to be clear, we've still got a loooong way to go, and I'm going to keep pushing. There's no rest for the weary as they say!

It seemed like almost instantly upon my feet hitting the LA soil (or concrete), Hollywood came knocking. Without even trying to put myself out there, casting agents and directors began reaching out: "I'm currently casting a TV show with a blind female lead. I love your content and personality and think you'd be perfect for the role! Would you be open to sending in an audition?"

While I had long since given up on my actress aspirations, that little girl with those big dreams still lived inside of me somewhere, and she was JUMPING for joy at the idea, so I did it for her. There was also some piece of me that was optimistic that if I could book a role as a blind character, I could also help mold that character into a more authentic portrayal and further my mission of increased (and authentic) representation.

Well, I must have done a pretty good job with my self-tape because... "We'd like to invite you to the studio to do a second read for the writer and producers." ME! MEEE! I was going to Studio City to audition for a major network television show.

Of course, it wouldn't be right if I didn't have a total blind girl moment the day of my big audition. My nails were well overdue for a manicure, and I simply couldn't go to my audition without getting them done because surely I wouldn't get the role with chipped nails. THAT would make or break the audition. I ran across the street to my typical salon and had my mom help pick out the perfect pastel pink-nude shade. Simple, clean, sophisticated, and unassuming, perfect for that stripped-back audition look. "She'll get shade ninety-six," my mom told the nail tech as she walked out.

Turns out that ninety-six and sixty-nine look very similar to sighted folks, because when I arrived home an hour later and revealed my new nails to my mom, she was shocked by what she saw. "Did you ask for that? Did you change colors after I left?" What was she talking about? I was so confused. "They're neon pink..." she informed me. Of course, I had no idea and had happily paid and walked home without knowing.

We raced back over and discovered how the mix-up happened. "Can you fix them?" we asked in a panic. And they did... but it turns out my cuticles can only handle so much acetone soaking before they begin to bleed. Peeling nail beds and painful fingertips aside, my perfectly nude nails and I were ready to impress.

"Oh my god! Hi! Can I give you a hug? I feel like I already know you!" Things were off to a good start as I entered the small, tightly packed audition room. "I'm so glad you agreed to audition! I watched all of your YouTube videos when writing this show! I hope I did it justice!"

The main character's name was Murphy, she went blind at fourteen from retinitis pigmentosa, and she had a guide dog. I'm blind, but even I could see the similarities. The guide dog was named Pretzel, a name I remember mentioning on YouTube when talking about my favorite guide dog.

She laughed out loud as I performed with as much confidence and charisma as I could muster. "Good. Can we do it again with a little more sass?" one woman piped up.

"Yeah, of course, no problem!"

After three or four takes, I turned to exit the room, when the writer said, "I really hope you get the role. If not, we'll definitely hire you to consult on set."

Spoiler alert, a sighted girl got the role, and I was not hired to consult. This began a long road of random requests for auditions. I found myself getting through round after round, down to the finals time and time again, only to lose it to a sighted actress who could obviously play a more convincing blind person than me. (Eye roll.) Just like with any job, when sighted or non-disabled people are the ones doing the hiring, it's easier for them to pick what they know than to challenge themselves to work with someone who may have different needs from what they're used to.

After years of hope and disappointment, I finally decided to give up. "I love what I do, I don't need to be in movies or on TV to be happy. I'm done wasting my time trying." I told my mom this after she finished reading the next audition opportunity that landed in our inbox.

"Good, I'll just ignore it, then," she said, putting her phone down.

Three times. They reached out three times through every avenue possible. I told them no, but they kept pushing. I finally agreed to get on a call with the casting agent, and she told me, "The producers really want you and they're willing to do anything to make it happen. They'll adjust the filming schedule around when you're available and will make sure to get all your scenes done as quickly as possible." She went on to explain that they'd give me a higher rate than the average series regular, and a higher title too. "It would be great for your career!" she tried to convince me.

"Fine. I'll do it next week when I'm home." I was on a trip in Japan and in no rush to get it done. If they wanted me that bad, they could wait until I was ready. I was done bending over backward to make it happen, knowing this would probably end with the same fate as every other audition before it.

Jet-lagged by the seventeen-hour time change, I somehow managed to memorize my lines. "I don't want to do this," I said to my dad as we practiced.

"Just give it a shot—you've already got the script down."

I was tired. I had only arrived home twelve hours prior, and I was leaving the next morning for yet another work trip. I knew this wouldn't be my best, so why waste my time? We all knew I wasn't going to get it anyway.

"You don't know that! They seem to reaaallyyyyyy want you this time," my mom reminded me.

A few quick takes down, I sent off the best options with no expectations. But when I landed after my flight the next day, I received an email.

These are really good! A little stiff at times but a solid audition overall. I'll let you know when I hear something.

I appreciated the feedback, and given the casting agent had seen all the other auditions, I felt like this was a good sign.

BUUTTT then they dragged me along for months. I was told, "They loved you, they're just waiting until they cast the lead before they cast the character you're up for." The producers even offered me another single episode role in one of their other shows, but the shooting conflicted with my schedule. "I mean, if they want to cast me in another one of their shows, I think that's a good sign! They obviously think I'm decent enough, right?" I said to my parents, feeling quite confident.

Then I got the message: **It was between you and two other girls, and they decided to go with someone else. They didn't give a reason.** CLASSIC. Just what I expected. How could I even be surprised or disappointed at this point?

The main character's last name was Burke, and she was slowly going blind due to a degenerative disease. The role I was up for was a young girl in her twenties named Mia who has a guide dog and went blind in her teens but has a sunny, positive attitude and works to help uplift other blind people. The writers followed me on Instagram, and once again, the inspiration was clear.

I tried not to be bitter, just happy that my content had been a source of motivation to create more blind characters in media and could provide some insight on what real blindness can be like. But, it's hard to not be a little salty when things like this happen:

My mom and I had finished sifting through the latest Free People collection and were about to leave when . . .

"Excuse me. I'm sorry... are, are you Molly Burke?"

I'm used to strangers approaching me to say hi, or even take a picture. I love having a chance to stop and chat with my followers, so I turned with a smile on my face. "Hi! Yes, I am!"

"Oh my god, no way. This is crazy! I'm a stylist and I'm currently working on a project with blind characters!"

"Wow—that's so cool! Do you mind me asking what it is?"

"Well, actually, it's a TV show, and the character is kind of based off of you!" she replied, not seeming to realize the bomb she'd dropped, but my heart utterly sank. **Are you kidding me? This can't be happening again.** "I'm actually shopping for the character right now. Is there anything here you think I should pick up?"

"Well, you came to the right store." I was trying so hard to sound nonchalant. **Did she really just ask me that?** "This IS my style!" I said, gesturing to my outfit, which was purchased from this very establishment. **It has to be. It has to be the same show. I need to hear her say it.** "I'd love to hear more about it..." I trail off. My mouth felt dry.

She told me the name of the show. **Yep. That's it.**

"Huh, that's so ironic. I actually auditioned for that but I just found out I didn't get the part." I was trying my best to casually play it off like it was no big deal.

But this was definitely her **oh shit** moment. She knew she'd put her foot in her mouth but dug the hole deeper. "Oh! I didn't even know you auditioned... I mean, you're the inspiration for the character," she reiterated awkwardly.

Trying to keep the same smile on my face, I assured her, "As long as the person who was cast is actually blind, I'll be happy, because that's what matters most: authentic representation." It was true, but I couldn't help feeling pissed off. Even if they had hired a blind person, this character was apparently inspired by me—**Am I not good enough to play myself?**

"Seriously. How has this happened again?!" Frustrated, I bitched to my mom as we continued to walk around the mall. "I mean, I obviously had a feeling based on the audition sides and character breakdown, but I'm not conceited enough to say that for sure I inspired this character, but now... now I know for sure, and now I'm really frustrated and want to know why they didn't pick me. If they had their doubts, give me feedback, give me another audition, have me do a read with the lead... What happened?" I ranted. "This story is definitely going in my book!" "Yes, exactly, Molly. Now you have a great story for your book." (And here we are, it made the book!)

"Text the casting agent. Tell her what we found out," I demanded as we stood in line to pay for the squeaky toy my new guide dog, Elton, had just picked out. With a little hesitation, she typed out the message on her phone as I dictated it to her. That text led to this email (for legal reasons, I can't give you the whole email verbatim, so I will paraphrase where necessary):

"Casting just followed up with me today about this incident. They feel so bad." They seemed to think my problem was the unprofessionalism of the stylist, who they assured me was simply a junior assistant buyer, which was in no way the issue. I was told the two producers wanted to profusely apologize to me, but "the character is not Molly, and was not written based on Molly." They said the assistant must have been mistaken, that she was starstruck and overexpressed herself. "Perhaps the assistant may have seen a photo of Molly on the wall when the stylist was putting together looks, as Molly is an influencer, and she is known for her fun style and looks." I call BS. While I wish I were simply known as a fashion guru on social media, I'm well aware that isn't my niche. There are many fashion girlies who are known for their style, but if you ask someone what they know me for, it's most likely for being blind.

They reiterated that they thought the assistant's actions were inappropriate and that they spoke to her about it. The way it was written made it sound like she got reprimanded. I found it very upsetting because that wasn't my intention, and her behavior had never been the problem. What she did would only be "inappropriate" if the character actually was based on me, and I didn't get the part. If I had gotten the part, of course they would want my opinion on the wardrobe, and if it wasn't based on me, then my opinion wouldn't be relevant anyway.

They went on to ask if we could work together to promote the show, "somehow on her socials, or include her somehow in another way?" They ended by, for the fifth time in one email, profusely apologizing.

I'm sure they're "very sorry" they got caught, I thought to myself after reading it. **You don't have to apologize a million times if you're not guilty.** And the way they suggested we find other avenues to work together made it feel like they were trying to buy my silence.

Maybe it was just my own wounded view of things, but I couldn't help but feel unconvinced by this response to getting called out. Following this, I noticed there was a name change to one of the blind characters. While her last name was originally Burke in early press, it no longer was when the show came out. Coincidence? You decide for yourself.

I try to remind myself that increased representation is what my goal has always been, even if I don't get to be involved. "You should be flattered! You're helping people create strong, confident blind characters!" my mom always tells me. While I try to be grateful and flattered, I am also human and that comes with all sorts of complicated and conflicting emotions. I no longer trust Hollywood. I stick to what clearly works for me: speaking, content creation, and advocating for change behind the scenes so that others can have their moment in the spotlight.

These are just two notable experiences of many. I've auditioned countless times for many other blind characters in shows and movies, getting down to the final rounds of auditions and losing (but hey, maybe I'm just a bad actor). These roles used to ALWAYS go to a sighted person, but now they just SOMETIMES do! And that brings me hope. Progress is progress, and I can get behind that!

What I can't get behind is when elements of me, my story, my likeness, and my characteristics, are ripped off by writers and producers. It's frustrating and screams, **We aren't hiring inclusively**; no blind writer, director, producer, and maybe not even a blind actor, so the easiest thing to do is use a real blind person to inform the character. They can watch hours upon hours of my content—over two thousand videos that I've posted on different platforms throughout the years. I've given them everything they need. For free.

To be clear, I don't have a problem with creatives using my content to help learn about my community. That's why I started making content to begin with. But it's important to remember that I am just one blind person sharing one lived experience. It should be supplementary to hiring inclusively so that my content isn't the one data point they are using. In reality, if I am one of the only ways these people are learning about blindness, then their representation of blindness is still inauthentic because it's all based on one person and not the diversity of our actual community. Representation isn't just important on screen, it's important at every level to truly do justice by a minority group. As the disability community always says, "Nothing about us without us."

THE FACE OF BLINDNESS

In the same way that I don't feel represented by media's portrayal of blindness, some blind people don't feel represented by me. I was scrolling my Twitter when I stumbled upon a thread:

> She'll never be independent or be able to live alone, she needs her mom to do everything for her.
>
> **Well, that's ridiculous. I lived on my own at eighteen.**
>
> She said she needs help knowing if she's on her period, are you kidding me? Ridiculous. You should be able to feel it and just know.
>
> **You know when you're on your period because you can "just feel it"? Great, I'm so glad for you, but I can't and why isn't that ok?**
>
> She's such a joke...an embarrassment to the blind community.

Surely, somebody's going to defend me.

I hope no one ever thinks I'm like her just because I'm also blind.

How much more are they going to say?

I felt my heart rate surging more with every tweet I read... but kept scrolling uncontrollably. I read about how much the very people I'd been trying to help were disappointed in me. And at least half the things they were saying weren't even true! What had I done wrong? I couldn't figure it out. All I'd ever wanted to do was uplift my community, and nothing could be more devastating than finding out I had failed them. It was earth-shattering. I saw the blatant hypocrisy in their words; as a community we constantly shout that we are not a monolith, that despite all living with vision loss, we are not the same, yet they were acting like I should be. We're all allowed to accommodate ourselves in different ways that make sense for our lives. If we are asking others outside of our community to treat us as individuals, then we ourselves need to do so. If we want non-disabled people to respect us and stand with us, we need to be united in our messaging, regardless of our differences. Even though I knew this, it still hurt and was frustrating that others didn't see it this way, but I guess that's the point—we're all different.

This went deeper than "haters"—hate comments had never gotten to me in this way. This was more than just "bullying"—I had learned to overcome and live above the bullying. This felt like the biggest betrayal in my life to date, and I hate to admit it, but it got to me. It messed with my mind and my self-esteem for a long time, and it took a lot of therapy to come to terms with it. Even now I still feel fearful when I meet other blind people: **Are they one of the ones I've disappointed? Do they hate me? Do they believe these things that are being said about me?**

But as I worked through my emotions surrounding this, I ended up connecting with other blind people in the public eye who have had similar experiences and faced the same judgments and backlash. It helped me to realize that it's not just ME. I'm not really the problem here at all. Once I realized other blind people went through something similar, a weight was lifted off my shoulders. I could breathe again.

Social media was a way for me to take back MY voice and MY story from the mainstream media, but as my platform grew and I noticed that I was the only disabled creator really "making it," I started to feel an immense pressure or even an obligation to try to represent my community as a whole. It didn't matter how many times I reminded people, "I'm just one blind person and this is how I do it," or "I don't represent all blind people," I knew that with me and my content being the only "real blind person" many people were ever exposed to, I had accidentally become the face of blindness.

It felt lonely. I was never in it for ME to succeed; I was in it for my community to succeed. Now that I knew I had let them down, or at least some of them, I could go back to just being Molly again. Somehow, finding out that people don't like you is incredibly freeing. It gives you permission to stop trying to make them happy and focus on making yourself happy instead.

I've come to terms with the fact that I will never please everyone with who I am or what I do. Just like the saying goes, "You can be the ripest, sweetest peach, but some people just don't like peaches." And I'd like to add to that, some people are allergic to them, and that's okay. They aren't your people, they aren't your audience, so don't create for them; create for you and those who DO feel seen and heard by you. Some people in the blind community hate me, and I'll never change their minds; others love and support me, and tell me I've made a really positive impact on their lives. I no longer have time or energy to give to those who don't like me, even though their voices may echo louder. I choose to be the person I needed but never had, and that girl will resonate with whoever she's meant to.

I've spent too much of my life apologizing for who I am and trying to fit inside a box that wasn't built for me. I no longer want to be in a box, because there's way more space to play outside of it. My new motto is "Break the rules (but not the law) and be the square peg in the round hole." Life is so much more fun that way.

ALL FOR ONE AND ONE FOR ALL

As you've probably noticed by now, there have been so many times in my life when I've felt like I didn't fit in. That whole square-peg-round-hole situation has been basically just me my entire life. I mean, I quite literally live in a world that wasn't made for people like me. I, like many disabled people, have to constantly adapt, accommodate, and find work-arounds to get daily tasks done independently. It's taught me that independence looks different for everyone, disabled or not. However, as disabled people we often feel a deep internal pressure to be overachievers to combat the low expectations society has for us. We often have to work ten times harder to accomplish something in the hopes that others will view us as capable, or better yet, equal.

We're so wrapped up in a vicious cycle where our ableist society projects its limiting beliefs on our disabled children. This is how internalized ableism manifests. When I was younger, and first coming to terms with my vision loss, I was deeply entrenched in the medical model of disability, the most prolific out of the many schools of thought that exist around disability. It suggests that people with disabilities are broken, and that science and medicine can fix us. They want to heal us, to change us, so that we fit into society better. How could I not hold these beliefs for myself when I'd spent so many of my formative years working with a charity whose main goal was to cure retinal blindness? Charities like these create sob stories and pity parties out of children like me. **How sad, this poor little girl will never grow up to see her own face looking back at her in the mirror. She'll never be able to pick out her own wedding dress or see her child smile.** Their goal is to make you feel bad so that you want to donate money, but how do you think those words will translate into the minds of those of us living with these (currently incurable) diseases?[15] When I went blind, I thought I was worthless and wouldn't be able to live a happy, successful, fulfilling life because of cure culture and the medical model. I now believe that waiting for a cure that may never come is not living. You're putting your life on hold instead of diving headfirst into building the best life possible. It's about accepting what you cannot change, and focusing on what you can.

I've learned in my life that bad things happen (I think that's pretty clear at this point! Haha) but the worst thing you can do is to let it stop you. If I had stayed stuck in the grief of my

---

15. To be clear, I'm not against all medical research—I'm against the way charities and doctors position its importance. Basically, I have a bone to pick with their marketing team. It's also frustrating to see how much money gets poured into medical advancements that will take longer and help fewer people than increased accessibility will. If we allocate a bit more of that funding to supporting infrastructure changes to make the world more universally inclusive, it will go a long way.

vision loss, I'd never be where I am today: writing this **New York Times** number-one-bestselling book. (I'm manifesting here... fingers crossed!) As I came to accept myself, I realized that my blindness contributes to the whole person I am, and I love that person... flaws and all.

I now follow the social model. I no longer think that I am broken or not enough because of my blindness. I am simply different from a non-disabled person. Just like how a blonde is different from a brunette. It is the barriers society has created that really make me disabled. My vision loss simply means I perceive the world differently from someone with 20/20 vision. And the real cure for all disabilities is actually universal design—the idea of designing for EVERYONE and not just for what the average person needs. One of the earliest examples of this is the "curb cut"—the smooth slope where the sidewalk meets the street. Originally designed for wheelchair users, now anyone riding a bike, pushing a stroller, or pulling a suitcase can benefit. A happy accident that taught us so much! Universal design is clearly an asset but when you bake it in from the beginning of the design process it can push the boundaries of creativity and innovation even further. While progress is being made, there is still so much work to do. Society has yet to hit the pivot point where accessibility and inclusivity are the expectation and not the exception.

When websites are designed with accessibility in mind and I can navigate them independently with my screen reader, I don't feel disabled. I don't even THINK about the fact that I can't see. But the opposite is equally true. When touch screens don't support screen readers or connect to accessible apps, I am made to feel disabled. And even more than that, I am made to feel invisible, like I don't matter, and it's dehumanizing.

I feel the purest form of joy when I come face-to-face with an accessible product or service for the first time. I feel seen, I feel heard, and I feel that I matter. Accessibility provides independence and dignity. It fosters an inclusive world that allows disabled people to thrive. Even now, I'm still experiencing basic forms of independence for the first time. A few years ago, I worked on a campaign with a chocolatier who made the first braille legend to navigate the chocolate box. I was finally able to pick which chocolate I wanted to eat, instead of waiting for someone to read the options and hand me my selection. The average person probably never even realizes how difficult simple things like this can be for those of us with disabilities.

I grew up with parents who really encouraged me to focus on the things I was good at and forget the rest; they reminded me that everyone has different talents, skills, abilities, and opportunities in life and that I don't have to be good at everything—I can work to be great at a few things. Not to toot my own horn, but I do think I've honed a few of my skills to a level of greatness (at least that's what my parents tell me!) while deciding to forgo other skills entirely, like cooking.

Yes, it's true: I'm in my early thirties, and I can't cook. I will say, it's not for a lack of trying. I've taken many a cooking class, and even took two years of home economics at the school for the blind. Even with access to specialized training, I still cannot be trusted in the kitchen. For a long time, I felt a deep sense of shame about this, especially as a woman. Sometimes people still judge me for it (like those blind people on Twitter... It bothers them more than it bothers me!). They act like I'm somehow making ALL blind people look less capable because I, one blind person, cannot cook. Meanwhile, they may not possess skills that I have, like doing a full face of makeup without a mirror. Sure, one of those things might be more important than the other, but I don't care. Let me do my makeup and order Uber Eats, damn it! Being able to cook might be an important form of independence for some blind people, but it clearly isn't for me. After all, I've come to find that some sighted, non-disabled people can't cook OR do their makeup, so I guess I'm not doing so bad after all!

Maybe cooking independently has never been that important to me, but my financial independence definitely has, which is way harder than just being able to make a cheesecake (I think?). Having my financial independence never meant wealth to me; it simply meant not having to rely on family, a romantic partner, or the government; sadly, a true privilege in the disability community given the unemployment statistics.

It was beyond my wildest dreams to be able to buy my first home in my late twenties. (Oh, how far that girl sleeping on a mattress on the floor has come!) I was even able to renovate it to be an accessible space where I can feel safe, comfortable, and independent. I really wanted to find a way to marry beauty and luxury with accessibility. For the most part, accessible design is overly utilitarian. It's often ugly, sterile, and cold. We're not used to seeing it done in a beautiful, interesting way. It's looked at as a necessity to meet building code, not as something that can actually add to your space, and I wanted to change that.

I'm confident that once my renovations were (FINALLY) complete, my space was even more aesthetically pleasing. There's texture everywhere, so even though I can't see the color on the walls or the pattern of the tile, I can feel it. (You'd LOVE my polka-dot black-and-white tile. It's to die for!) Layering so much texture and adding in unique lighting solutions has created a lot of visual interest. It's something people notice and comment on the moment they walk through my front door.

I have tons of smart products: smart appliances, smart blinds, smart TV, smart lighting, and even a smart fireplace.[16]

Organization is really important for me. If everything has a place, I'll always be able to find it! All the extra built-in storage we added ended up making the condo more functional for anyone who lives there.

---

[16]. Take a shot every time I say "smart"! Unless you're under twenty-one... then sip on water.

I'll be honest, when I experience little moments of accessibility for the first time, like picking out my own chocolate or being able to navigate my smart TV, I feel emotional and sometimes even cry.[17] Most people have never had to think about these things because they've always had the privilege of doing it on their own ... I can't wait for the day when that's my reality. When I no longer question the accessibility everywhere I go and with everything I buy.

Unfortunately, a lack of accessibility is still something that's far too common in my day-to-day life. Every time I leave the comfort and safety of my home, I'm entering the unknown. **Will this crosswalk be accessible? Will the elevator buttons have braille? Will it say the floor number out loud? Does this touch screen have screen reader capabilities? Will I be able to do this on my own, or will I need to ask for help?** A product or service being inaccessible to me as a blind person is just one small, subtle way the world says, **Oops, we forgot about you.** Or even worse, **you don't matter to us.** The fact is, inaccessibility IS discrimination. We usually think of discrimination as an active choice, but passive behaviors can be just as damaging. And there's no reason that in this day and age this should still be an issue. It's time for change, and I'm not going to shut up about it until designing for all users is the standard.

---

17. Which says a lot, because I'm not a big crier.

LOUDMOUTH

I once read a comment on one of my videos that lives rent-free in my mind and went a little something like this:

> **My two-year-old son is blind, and I used to love your channel, but I unsubscribed once you started becoming really successful. I felt uncomfortable seeing someone with a disability making so much money and having so many big opportunities, it didn't feel fair or right. One day I stopped to think about it, and I realized how messed up that is. I felt uncomfortable because I had never seen a successful disabled person who had accomplished more than I, a sighted person, have. But I'm back now and I'm glad I am. I and my son SHOULD have a successful disabled person to look up to like you. Thank you!**

It really made me stop and think.

We need everyone to see disabled people thriving so that they believe it's possible and raise their disabled children to believe it's possible too. For that reason, I will not apologize for my luxury home, I will not apologize for my designer handbag (and now, I buy the handbag I actually love, not just the one that all the Instagram girls have—progress!), and I will not apologize for my sass. Maybe this sass is exactly what society needs to wake the fuck up.

In March of 2020, right before the world shut down, I spoke at an event in NYC for International Women's Day as a part of my Aerie contract. On a panel of seven women, my question came last. I was expecting something deep and meaningful, thought-provoking, something that would allow for me to provide an insightful answer like the other girls, but then I was hit with, "Tell us about your dating life—are you swiping on Bumble?"

Ah yes, the moderator needed to plug the sponsor of the panel, Bumble, the app where women message first, and with no one left but me, I was stuck with talking about my less-than-thrilling love life. Well, throw me under the bus and I'll pull you down with me. "No, I haven't personally found that app to be easy to use with my screen reader. So while I love their female empowerment angle, I don't think you can really consider something empowering unless it's empowering for everyone. I use Tinder instead because even though it's not perfect, it's easier for me to navigate with my screen reader. I encourage others to do the same or use other apps until it is more accessible for all users. I know there are some folks here from Bumble, so I'd love to chat about how to be more accessible moving forward after the panel!" The audience erupted into supportive cheers and applause, but you could feel the tension radiating off of the Bumble team sitting in the front row. I gave them the callout to come find me, but shockingly, they never took me up on it. I can't say whether or not they've changed their ways and made the app more screen reader-friendly because I've sworn off the apps since then, but if not, the offer still stands.

Reflecting back on this moment, some would say I stuck my foot in my mouth, but I still don't regret it. Just a few months later, Aerie would choose not to renew my contract for year three (though I'm like...98 percent sure the whole Bumble thing didn't have anything to do with it), and as devastating as it was, I know I left my mark, and most importantly, I did it with integrity. Early on in my career I had to rub shoulders, play by the rules, try to fit the mold, and smile, even in the face of injustice or ableism. I didn't have the power to speak up because I was still earning my right to be there. You can't make change if you aren't in the room, and you won't stay in the room long if you kick up a fuss before you've proven yourself and gained the respect of the gatekeepers. Even just a few years prior, I would have NEVER had the confidence to call out a brand like that, especially when I'm being paid to be there. But the new me knows that I've carved my path, and I've made my way to a position of power and privilege. And with that, I must take a stand for what I believe in and push for the change that I want to see in the world. I must speak for those who still aren't in the room, and I must stand behind my message one hundred percent, no matter what.

One hundred percent means one hundred percent of the time. I'm no longer here to be liked, I'm here to make change. And sometimes in order to make change, you have to be honest, which can make people uncomfortable. It forces them to do some self-reflection, and we don't always like what we're looking at, no matter how good our makeup is.

As you know by now, makeup has always been a love of mine. All things beauty and fashion—it's in my genes, just like RP (or should I say, jeans). I loved makeup before I knew I'd one day no longer be able to see it (yes, I was that little girl sneaking off to play with her mom's lipstick at the bathroom counter). The OG beauty gurus brought me to social media as a viewer, and as my platform eventually grew, I fantasized that I'd one day get to work with the same big brands as them. But no matter how much beauty-related content I made, they never came knocking. And when we knocked on their doors, they'd slam them in our faces. "She's not a makeup artist" was a common excuse, as if all the other content creators they'd worked with were (spoiler, they weren't).

All the reasons they gave felt like code for **she can't see the product to review it**. Which, yes, is entirely accurate. I can't do the average beauty review and tell you the exact color composition, how much coverage it has, or if it oxidizes throughout the day, but that's never what I was proposing. I wanted to go beyond the surface level that the industry is so often tied to and get to the root of what makeup is really all about. Not being able to see the makeup doesn't mean that I, like the average beauty lover and consumer, can't fully experience the most important parts of it. Self-care and self-expression are the true essence of what makes us love makeup, and that's something I can speak to on an even deeper level than most.

I don't and never have done my makeup to hide my acne scars or freckles, to look more beautiful, or even to feel more confident. I'm in a unique position in that I don't really know what I look like; therefore, I don't know the difference that concealer or a great volumizing mascara makes to my face. Makeup doesn't make me like myself more, and it's not something I do because I feel societal pressure to—it's something I do because I genuinely enjoy it. I enjoy taking time for myself every day to do something I love, and I enjoy playing with textures, colors, and styles to reflect how I'm feeling inside. A bright red lip makes me feel like a powerful girl boss and a soft pink blush makes me feel extra feminine. I also enjoy a pop of coral when I'm feeling beachy and flirty. Or a glittery liner to be festive. These are the conversations I want to have about beauty and what I want the non-makeup-lovers of the world to know. The beauty industry doesn't have to be shallow or vain, and it isn't for many of us. Sadly, for me it seemed like these were conversations few in the business were interested in having.

Thankfully, **Allure** magazine was. Yes, the iconic "best in beauty" magazine saw the value I could bring to the industry when no others did. "They want to send a camera crew over to your apartment to film a video for their YouTube channel!" I could hear the excitement in my manager's voice. **We're finally breaking through.**

This felt like a once-in-a-lifetime opportunity. I couldn't mess this up. I knew I was putting a lot of pressure on myself, but you don't get do-overs in this biz. I'd spent days cleaning and organizing my beauty products, I'd hired my favorite makeup artist to get me all dolled up, and I'd tried on at least half of my closet to find the perfect fit for the occasion. If only the crew had been the right fit...

It was the day of, and a team of four non-makeup-wearing men arrived, equipment in hand. They were mostly wearing black and making small talk while setting up. They seemed nice enough, but I was confused. I was expecting to have girlie time, getting to bond over beauty chats. But instead we were discussing the weather.

As I was sitting down at my vanity, the interview began with a jarring question "What's an eyebrow pencil?" and it quickly became apparent that the producer knew NOTHING about makeup. I knew this wasn't going to go well.

By the end of the shoot, I already knew I wouldn't be happy with the result, no matter how much editing they did. "Content geared toward a mainly female audience should be produced

BY women. At the very least, ONE of the men they sent should have been a makeup lover, but it was clear none of them knew anything about the subject we were discussing. They didn't know what questions to ask, so I didn't have a chance to talk about the things I think are important to discuss!" I ranted passionately on the phone to my manager. "Pull the plug. I don't want the video going out." I knew I was making myself seem difficult (not the reputation you want) and I was risking any future opportunities to work with **Allure**, but I didn't care. If it wasn't made in a way that I believed was right, I didn't want it to be seen, even if it could boost my career.

To my surprise, instead of rolling their eyes at me in dismay, **Allure** sent a giant box filled with every expensive beauty product I couldn't yet afford (think $500 Givenchy night cream) along with a long, apologetic email. **We agree with you. Please let us make this right.**

A week later, I jumped on a call with the new producer. I was a bit embarrassed, thinking this woman probably thought I was a diva for wanting to reshoot the piece. But instead, I was met with, "Thank you for what you did." She explained, "We've been having these discussions for a long time internally, pushing the higher-ups to have women making content for women, but they never listened. Most of the talent we work with come from a background of traditional media, so they're used to male-dominated sets and don't see anything wrong with it. But it took you, a talent our team respects, calling them out on it to make change. I can assure you that the entire crew for our next shoot with you will be women or people who wear makeup, but the shift is far beyond that. You speaking up has already created a ripple effect, and we're finally seeing more women getting the opportunities they've long deserved."

Hanging up the phone I knew I was finally done with my people-pleasing ways and avoiding confrontation. In that moment of intense frustration, I was overcome with enough emotion to not worry about what people would think, say, or do but rather to only be concerned by what I felt was an injustice. And the end result was not the negativity or backlash I feared but rather positive progress. I vowed from then on that I'd never let my morals or core values take a back seat and I'd use my loud mouth to scream for change from the rooftops. Sometimes it works out, and other times it doesn't. Sometimes it's intentional, and other times, it just comes out of me like an uncontrollable explosion of passion. Like when I received the Clio Health Award for my years of online advocacy and public speaking.

I sat in the audience watching the other winners accept their awards and was struck by how inaccessible the content was. So many of these winning ads were ABOUT disability and featured disabled people, yet none of them had audio description or captions. I had no idea what was happening the whole time. My mom sat next to me in the front row, describing things to me in my ear. We might've looked rude, but she was just trying to include me. My award was the final one of the evening, and as I practiced my speech in my head, I just knew I'd go off course once I got up there. **I might not say the right thing that people want to hear, but maybe that's exactly why I'm being honored.**

I had to take my chance while I had it because who knew when a moment like this would happen again. Speaking to a room of successful, talented advertising execs who hold so much power, I needed to remind them of what to do with it. I wasn't too sure how it would land, but after making my way through my memorized acceptance speech, I went rogue. "This wasn't planned, but it wouldn't be true and authentic to myself and my mission if I didn't take the opportunity in front of a room of complete changemakers like you to ask you to please think about adding audio description and captions to your content. Tonight, there've been so many beautiful ads shared, and most of it I could not consume because I didn't understand what was happening on the screen. So please consider the people who you're creating for—my community, disabled and chronically ill people, we need captions and we need audio description to be able to actually perceive the messages that you're sharing. They are so important, and believe me, there are ways to keep the integrity and the beauty of the art of the ads you are making while still being inclusive of my community."

I was nervous about it, but I hadn't shut my mouth because I felt like I was lucky to be there and needed to impress anyone.

I didn't worry that they'd be offended or take away my award. I did what I believed was right because I knew that I couldn't expect others to do something if I myself was unwilling to. I won because of my advocacy work, and that work isn't a job I clock in and clock out of—it's every day, it's every moment, it's my life. Speaking up, whether it's well received or not, is not just a onetime thing now. It's an every-chance-I-get thing, and I'm proud of how far I've come in finding my voice. The same voice that other people silenced, I now use with confidence and conviction. And sometimes I lose opportunities because I won't shut up, but that just means that it wasn't for me, it wasn't genuine or didn't authentically align with my values, so I wouldn't have really wanted it anyway. The right ones, like **Allure**, and the many attendees at that awards ceremony who came up to me the rest of the night, saying I completely changed their view and how they'd approach projects in the future, appreciate that I take every chance I get to speak my truth with passion, and they invite it.

Thanks to **Allure** giving me their vote of confidence, I've been able to partner with a number of forward-thinking skin-care, makeup, and hair-care brands who want to strive for greater inclusivity. I've continued to work with the **Allure** team, including being featured in an editorial piece in their print magazine and filming more video content. My favorite was when I got to work with them on reviewing the accessibility of different beauty products. That viral video opened an entire new career path for me, corporate consulting on product packaging, universal design, and inclusive marketing. But perhaps the most meaningful gift **Allure** gave me was awarding me with the title of **Allure** A-Lister. At the inaugural event in 2022, I was honored as one of the nineteen faces "changing the beauty industry." No, I couldn't believe it either.

As I stood on the rooftop of the Pendry Hotel, cocktail in hand, I took the moment to reflect on how hard it had been to get there. In my black Prada loafers, Pleats Please pants, and that bold red lip, I was my very own "it girl." I felt the cool evening air fill my lungs and enjoyed the electric buzz of the celebration around me. I thought about the fourteen-year-old version of me, sitting on her black-and-white-striped duvet, eyeliner in hand, wondering if she'd ever feel okay again. The one who'd watch makeup tutorial after makeup review after makeup haul, just wishing to be as confident and successful as those creators she loved so much. This was more than an award to win or title to hold: it was a full-circle moment. **And I am so damn proud.**

EPILOGUE

Life is full of duality. It's what makes it so complex, but also what makes it so interesting. I think of myself as two distinctly different people. There's the Molly before vision loss and the Molly after, with the most life-altered version of me living somewhere in between. I only wish I could go back and tell that girl that all the no's, every setback, the hardships and failures, were really just lessons in disguise, preparing her and pushing her forward. And that one day, she'd take all that pain and create more purpose than she could have ever hoped for. But hey, I guess she didn't need to hear it; whether she knew it or not, she had the strength all along. And I want to thank her for everything she's done for me.

Before vision loss, I was so bubbly and precocious. Despite the difficult moments I faced, I was somehow still so carefree. For a long time, I wanted that girl back. She was innocent and naïve to the world. But I no longer miss her, and I no longer need her. I'm confident who I am is who I was always meant to be.

The ups and downs that are true to my journey have continued. A toxic relationship, losing not one but two more guide dogs, my dad's job loss, and my mom's skin cancer scare. The hard stuff keeps happening, but so does the good. A new boyfriend who helps heal every wound the last one left. Meeting my fourth guide dog, a beautiful fluffy boy named Elton, who's writing his very own children's book! Seeing my brother getting married and buying his first home with the most wonderful sister-in-law a girl could ask for. My parents both healthy and happy, working alongside me to keep this whole thing going! Continuing to be accused of faking blind but still getting to speak about accessibility at the World Economic Forum in Davos, Switzerland. Losing yet another movie role, but gaining another title: **Forbes** 30 Under 30.

All of these things coexist and are a part of what makes every day an adventure. Some days are higher than high, others are lower than low. And others fall somewhere in between. The hard parts of life are undeniably hard, but they also keep me driven.

I've lived many lives in my thirty years, but I think you could sum all of them up with just one word: "bittersweet." There have been seasons in my life that have been painful, traumatic, and even downright cruel. But it's also been beautiful, inspiring, and more magical than I could have ever imagined. I don't know if I'm cursed or if I'm blessed—I've certainly felt both at times. One thing I know for sure, though, is that you can't enjoy the full breath of sweetness without a little taste of the bitter. And you can never truly be seen until you see yourself for who you really are.

UNSEEN

I spent so much of my life feeling unseen. Unseen by my peers who saw my disability before they saw me. Unseen by society, by people who assume I'm training my service dog for someone else, or who ask my boyfriend what I'm going to order for lunch instead of asking me. Unseen by developers, designers, and marketing agencies who don't realize that blind people buy and use products too. Unseen by an industry I love but that's so focused on perfection, it forgets that authenticity is better than perfect will ever be. Even unseen by some of my own community, who criticized the way that I chose to accommodate myself. I spent years trying to be seen as someone I'm not because being seen as a made-up version of me felt better than being invisible. Sometimes I'm still unseen, and all I can do is use my voice, speak up, and force them to notice, to understand: to care.

I think we all feel a little invisible sometimes, and maybe sometimes that's what we want. Blending in can feel easier, but I promise you, standing out is way more fun. I found the success I have by creating a space where there was none and being the fullest, most unapologetic version of Molly.

Sometimes I look back at my life and ask myself, **How did I survive? How did I get through it?** We as humans are far more resilient than we give ourselves credit for. When life hands you an unimaginably heavy weight to bear, you find an inner strength that you didn't know you had. I didn't just "get through" things: I pushed, I fought, I hoped, I cried (a lot),

I believed, and I overcame. We all have to overcome challenges time and time again. Some are big, some are small. For some it's often, and others it's rare. But no matter what, your adversity is valid.

I used to hope that I'd just hit my midlife crisis extra early, and I was done with hardship, but the harsh reality is that it's never done. There will always be lessons we don't really want to learn but are grateful we did, and there will always be moments where we don't know how we're going to survive, but we do and are better because of it.

I wouldn't wish my hardships on my worst enemy, not even Marissa, Dick, or the internet haters. I can't say I'd go back and do it all again (and PLEASE, GOD, don't make me!). But I also wouldn't trade it in for a different life either. Without the bitter, there'd be no sweet, and the sweetness in my life has been cavity-inducing. The bitter pain gave me sweet purpose, and that's just the way I see it.

GLOSSARY

Hey, friend, Molly here again! I'm currently cozied up in bed in one of my classic, go-to onesies with a soy latte in hand and Elton John lying on the floor beside me (the dog, not the person). I hope you're enjoying my story so far. I assume you've found yourself here at the back of the book because you're a little confused by something, and that's why the glossary is here! That said, please keep in mind that I don't claim to be an expert in anything except my own life. I am speaking for me and me alone. I am sharing my experiences, perspective, and ideas, and the knowledge I've gained and beliefs I hold. I do not represent the entire blind community, because no one person ever could, just like you don't represent all redheads or all tall people. We are a community as diverse as any other, and I refuse to bear the burden of being THE blind spokesperson because I'm just Molly, a girl who happens to be blind. And you're just Ryan, a guy who happens to be tall and have red hair. (Sorry, Ryan, didn't mean to single you out!)

I've shared my life online for the past decade, and I know that my thoughts, feelings, and opinions have changed over time. Just because twenty-two-year-old me said something doesn't mean that thirty-year-old me agrees, and thirty-six-year-old

GLOSSARY

me might not agree with everything my current self says in the pages to come. So, to be crystal clear, this book contains my perspective and ideas as of the time that I'm writing it. If you're reading this in 2042, well... some things have probably changed, or at least I'd like to hope they have, because personal growth is pretty damn important. All right, disclaimer over!

Okay, it's time to stop rambling on as I'm known to do sometimes and get on with it. In no particular order...

Guide Dog—Everyone loves dogs, so this seems like a good place to start! (At least, everyone SHOULD love dogs.) A guide dog is a specific type of service dog that is used by blind or visually impaired people. You may have heard of them referred to as "seeing-eye dogs," but that would be incorrect. Using that term is like using a brand name versus a product type. Basically, my guide dog is the generic-brand seeing-eye dog, but trust me, he wasn't any cheaper.

White Cane—A white cane specifically refers to a mobility aid that is used by a person who is blind or has low vision. All white or white and red are the most common, but the colors can actually symbolize different things depending on which country you're in. For example, in America all white means total blindness, and white and red means low vision, but in Canada everyone uses a white-and-red cane regardless of their level of vision loss, and in the UK all white is for blindness, and white and red is for deaf-blindness. You may also see custom canes in a variety of colors and even glitter! Yes, I do in fact have a hot pink AND a glitter cane. Although "white cane" is the more official name, we in the blind community typically just call it a cane, so that's probably how you'll see me refer to it.

Orientation and Mobility—Orientation and mobility, or O&M for short, is the professional training we in the blind community receive to learn how to safely navigate, whether that be with a cane or guide dog, or without a mobility aid of any kind. (In fact, only an estimated 2–8 percent of blind people use a white cane and around 2 percent use a guide dog.) This training does include learning to hit people in the ankles when they make rude comments, so be careful, and always remember: We can't SEE... but most of us have great hearing.

Sighted Guide—Sighted guide is basically when a human becomes the guide dog! A blind person will hold on to the elbow of the person providing the sighted guide, and by walking about a step behind you, we can feel where you are going the same way we do through the guide dog's harness. (NEVER try to randomly hold our hand, or even worse, grab our shoulders from behind and push us forward to direct us.) There are some specific techniques to it, so if you'd like to learn how to do it, I encourage you to use that nifty little tool we all have at our fingertips called Google!

GLOSSARY

Retinitis Pigmentosa—Retinitis pigmentosa, or RP as we in the community often call it, is the rare genetic eye disease I was born with that causes progressive vision loss due to the deterioration of the retina. There is currently no known cure or treatment, at least not for my gene type (TULP1, for the one person reading this who may actually care to know). Don't worry, it might be genetic, but it is not contagious, so you will not catch it by standing next to me in line at the grocery store.

Nystagmus—Nystagmus is yet another rare disease I was born with (because I'm THAT lucky), and it causes my eyes to constantly shake. In my case, it's in a circular motion and is entirely involuntary. They are the life of the party and hence never stop dancing, no music required.

Legally Blind—Legal blindness is where the blind community begins; total blindness is where it ends. Blindness, like most things in life, is a spectrum. Fun fact, less than 10 percent of blind people are actually completely blind, meaning 90 percent have some form of remaining vision. To be considered legally blind in North America (which essentially means you don't see enough to be able to drive a car), you have to have 20/200 vision or less than twenty degrees of visual field (meaning your peripheral vision is not as wide, almost like you're looking through a toilet paper roll or even a straw). This is WITH best correction, so no, Karen, you aren't legally blind without

GLOSSARY

your glasses. The term "legally blind" quite literally means WITH glasses on.

Screen Reader—Yes, believe it or not the tech world has actually recognized that blind people exist and could be potential paying customers, SO on top of things like Siri, Alexa, and Google Assistant, they've come up with something called a screen reader. There are multiple types of screen readers, but I typically use VoiceOver and TalkBack the most, which are the Apple and Android screen readers that come preloaded on all of their devices. Using key commands on my laptop or hand gestures on my touch-screen phone, I'm basically able to do everything you can do on your device except, you know… see the screen. (Unless the app or website isn't screen reader compatible, aka not accessible or inclusive. We hate those.)

Braille—You know those little raised bumps you see on elevator buttons or bathroom doors? Well, these bumps actually serve a purpose! Braille is a tactile code made up of six dots that allow blind people like me to read with our fingers, which is pretty cool! (Side note, I really wish they wouldn't put it ON the door; beside the door would be much better, because it's pretty awkward trying to read the door when someone on the other side opens it, and potentially even dangerous!) And yes, it does mean that I could read a book in the middle of a blackout. Come to think of it, I can actually do a lot of things in a blackout

GLOSSARY

that sighted people probably couldn't. Fun fact: braille is not its own language; it is a code that can be translated into any language. It's actually the only code that can do this. There are even braille codes for music and math! How cool!

Vision Itinerant—A vision itinerant is a teacher that is specifically trained to work with the blind and low-vision community. They do things like teach braille, transcribe print into braille and vice versa, and help the general class teacher make school more accessible by coming up with reasonable accommodations for the blind student. An educational assistant, or EA, may also be utilized in the classroom to support a blind student when a vision itinerant isn't present. They offer more generalized one-on-one support to students with a variety of disabilities. With my level of vision loss, I qualified for 100 percent support, which means I had a vision itinerant in class with me for 50 percent of the time and an EA the other 50 percent. (Keep in mind that I was raised in Canada, so the terms may differ in other places!)

Ableism—Ableism is to disabled people what racism is to the BIPOC community or homophobia is to the gay community. Yes, we get our very own special word to describe the discrimination we face—fun! (I feel the need to specify that I'm saying this in a VERY sarcastic tone of voice.)

ACKNOWLEDGMENTS

I don't believe anyone can truly claim to be "self-made"; I certainly never would. No matter how much hard work I've put into being where I am today, there are so many people who have equally committed their time, energy, love, and support to enable me to reach my full potential in life, and with this book. So now, I think it's time to share the spotlight and give some much deserved thank-yous!

Courtney Paganelli, you deserve this first shout-out, because this book truly wouldn't exist without you. You have consistently gone above and beyond to show your dedication to this project and your belief in me. I don't know how I would have reached the finish line, or even started the race, without you cheering me on every step of the way. You've shared your wisdom, your heart, and you've held my hand through every hard moment and important decision. Thank you for choosing to go on this journey with me and showing what a real ally is. I hope this is our first book of many together!

To the Abrams team, thank you for helping me bring my words to the world. I appreciate your willingness to learn, be flexible, and collaborate to create something that we can all be proud of, knowing it's the most accessible, inclusive book

ACKNOWLEDGMENTS

we could produce. I hope this project has opened your eyes (pun intended) to new ways that you can continue to move the needle forward in making the literary experience more universally enjoyable.

Reuven Ashtar, you believed in me when no one in the industry did. Hell, you believed in me when not even I did. You are more than a manager to me, you are family. Thank you for trusting me, fighting for me, and for the eight years of hard but rewarding work. My success is your success, and here's to so much more of it!

Brady, you are undoubtedly the best big brother a girl could ask for. You have been everything I've needed, even when I didn't know it. It doesn't matter how old we get, I will continue to look up to you with admiration. I have always been and will always be SO proud to be your little sister. And Léa, thank you for being the sister-in-law of my dreams. You are the best addition to this family!

Brendan, thank you for being the partner I've needed throughout this project and in life. I love knowing that I always have you there to bounce ideas off of or to look up a word in the thesaurus.

Last, but certainly not least, my parents. Niamh and Peter, I quite literally wouldn't be here without you. There is no way to put into words my eternal gratitude for everything you are and everything you've been for me. I'll never know why I was so blessed to have parents as wonderful as you, but trust me,

ACKNOWLEDGMENTS

I know how lucky I am. I am who I am because of you, and "thank you" will never be enough. I love you, and I promise to continue to try and make you proud every day.

PS. I can't end these acknowledgments without a little shout-out to Elton John (the dog)! Thanks for sitting by my side during countless hours of writing, which I'm sure were incredibly boring for you. Perhaps even more than your guiding skills, I appreciate all of the hugs and laughter you provide me with during the hard times. You're truly one-of-a-kind and a special, fluffy little muppet! Now that this book is FINALLY done, I think we should celebrate by going shopping together and letting you pick out a new stuffed animal, what do ya say?!

ABOUT THE AUTHOR

Molly Burke is a multi-hyphenate creative and advocate—a blind public speaker, content creator, consultant, model, and author—who has built a powerful global platform of over five million followers. Through her work, she passionately advocates for inclusion and authentic representation, using storytelling to uplift and empower communities worldwide. Her voice has been heard on some of the most prestigious stages—from the United Nations to the World Economic Forum in Davos—and earned her an honorary Clio Health Award. Named to **Forbes 30 Under 30**, Molly has been profiled by **The Wall Street Journal, People, Paper, Adweek, Teen Vogue, Allure**, and **Forbes**, and has appeared on **The Daily Show with Trevor Noah** and **The Today Show**. She's partnered with some of the world's most recognizable brands, from fashion and beauty to tech and entertainment, including Aerie, Estée Lauder, Dove, Tommy Hilfiger, Crocs, Google, Microsoft, Samsung, Bose, and Disney, helping to redefine how companies approach accessibility and representation.